HIV
Infection

A CLINICAL APPROACH

MARY M. FANNING
M.D., Ph.D., F.R.C.P.C., F.A.C.P.

Associate Professor, Division of Infectious Diseases,
Department of Medicine
Georgetown University Medical Center
Washington, D.C.

SECOND EDITION

W.B. SAUNDERS COMPANY
A Division of Harcourt Brace & Company

PHILADELPHIA   LONDON   TORONTO
MONTREAL   SYDNEY   TOKYO

W.B. SAUNDERS COMPANY
A Division of Harcourt Brace & Company

The Curtis Center
Independence Square West
Philadelphia, Pennsylvania 19106

Library of Congress Cataloging-in-Publication Data

HIV infection : a clinical approach / [edited by] Mary M.
  Fanning. —2nd ed.
      p.   cm.
  Includes bibliographical references and index.
  ISBN 0-7216-2792-7
  1. HIV infections—Handbooks, manuals, etc. I.
  Fanning, Mary M.
  [DNLM: 1. HIV Infections.   WC 503 H674 1997]
RC607.A26H572   1997
616.97′92—dc20
DNLM/DLC   96-22874

HIV INFECTION   ISBN 0-7216-2792-7

Printed in the United States of America.

Last digit is the print number: 9   8   7   6   5   4   3   2   1

This book is dedicated to the memory of

Robert Van Dusen,

who lived bravely with AIDS and worked in partnership

with us throughout the development of the manual.

Robert's enthusiasm for life will never be forgotten.

iii

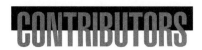
CONTRIBUTORS

Ian Barton, M.S.W.
HIV Social Work, Wellesley Health Centre, Toronto, Ontario, Canada

Psychiatric and Psychosocial Issues (HIV Team Approach)

Ahmed Bayoumi, M.D., F.R.C.P.C.
Clinical Fellow, The Wellesley Hospital, Toronto, Ontario, Canada

System- and Problem-Oriented Evaluation (Mycobacterium Avium Complex Infection)

Philip Berger, M.D., C.C.F.P., F.C.F.P.
Associate Professor, Department of Family and Community Medicine, Faculty of Medicine, University of Toronto; Chief, Department of Family and Community Medicine, The Wellesley Central Hospital, Toronto, Ontario, Canada

Heroin, Crack Cocaine, and HIV Infection (An Approach to Addicted HIV Patients)

Charles K.N. Chan, M.D., F.R.C.P.C., F.C.C.P., F.A.C.P.
Associate Professor of Medicine, Faculty of Medicine, University of Toronto; The Toronto Hospital, Toronto, Ontario, Canada

System- and Problem-Oriented Evaluation (Respiratory Manifestations), (Pneumocystis Carinii *Pneumonia*)

Brian Cornelson, M.D., C.C.F.P.
Assistant Professor, Department of Family and Community Medicine, Faculty of Medicine, University of Toronto; The Wellesley Central Hospital, Toronto, Ontario, Canada

HIV Primary Care Evaluation and Management (HIV Testing), (Medical Evaluation and Management)

Dale Dotten, M.D., F.R.C.P.C.
Associate Professor, Department of Medicine, University of Toronto; Head, Division of Hematology, The Wellesley Central Hospital, Toronto, Ontario, Canada

System- and Problem-Oriented Evaluation (Hematologic Manifestations)

Dianna Drascic, B.ScN., M.ScN.,/A.C.N.P.
McMaster University, Hamilton, Ontario; Clinical Nurse
Specialist/Acute Care Nurse Practitioner, HIV Services,
The Wellesley Central Hospital, Toronto, Ontario, Canada

Palliative Care and Pain Management

Mary Fanning, M.D., Ph.D., F.R.C.P.C., F.A.C.P.
Associate Professor, Division of Infectious Diseases,
Department of Medicine, Georgetown University Medical
Center, Washington, D.C.

*Introduction to HIV; An Approach to Patients with HIV
(Suggested Approach to Patients with HIV), (The Role of
Advocacy in Patient Care); HIV Primary Care Evaluation
and Management (Medical Evaluation and Management);
Heroin, Crack Cocaine, and HIV Infection (Medical
Complications of HIV in IV Drug Users); System- and
Problem-Oriented Evaluation (Fever), (Candida),
(Cytomegalovirus), (Herpes Simplex Virus), (Varicella-
Zoster Virus), (Histoplasmosis), (Tuberculosis)*

Joyce Fenuta, R.N.
Program Manager, Respirology, The Wellesley Central
Hospital, Toronto, Ontario, Canada

The Role of Nursing in HIV/AIDS Care

Benjamin K. Fisher, M.D., F.R.C.P.C.
Professor Emeritus, Department of Medicine
(Dermatology), University of Toronto, Medical School;
Chief, Division of Dermatology, The Wellesley Hospital,
Toronto, Ontario, Canada

*System- and Problem-Oriented Evaluation (Dermatologic
Manifestations)*

Michelle Foisy, Pharm.D.
Assistant Professor, Doctor of Pharmacy Program, The
University of Toronto; Clinical Pharmacist, Infectious
Diseases and General Medicine, The Wellesley Hospital,
Toronto, Ontario, Canada

*System- and Problem-Oriented Evaluation (Adverse Drug
Reactions in HIV Patients), (Drug Interactions in HIV
Patients); Adverse Effects of HIV Drugs: Incidence
and Management; Drug Desensitization Protocols;
Drug–Drug Interactions; Drug–Food Interactions*

Richard Fralick, M.D., F.R.C.P.
Assistant Professor, Department of Preventive Medicine
and BioStatistics, Department of Family and Community
Medicine; University of Toronto, The Wellesley Central
Hospital, Toronto, Ontario, Canada

*Heroin, Crack Cocaine, and HIV Infection (An Approach
to Addicted HIV Patients)*

Dafna Gladman, M.D., F.R.C.P.C.
Professor, Department of Medicine, University of Toronto;
Deputy Director, Centre for Prognosis Studies in Rheu-
matic Diseases, Toronto Hospital–Western Division,
Toronto, Ontario, Canada

*System- and Problem-Oriented Evaluation
(Musculoskeletal Complications)*

Mark H. Halman, M.D., F.R.C.P.C.
Lecturer of Psychiatry, University of Toronto; Director,
HIV Psychiatry Program, The Wellesley Central and Saint
Michael's Hospitals, Toronto, Ontario, Canada

*Psychiatric and Psychosocial Issues (Psychiatric
Disorders in HIV-Infected Individuals), (Psychotherapy
with HIV-Infected Individuals)*

Helen Harrison, R.N.
Clinical Co-ordinator, General Internal Medicine, The
Wellesley Central Hospital, Toronto, Ontario, Canada

The Role of Nursing in HIV/AIDS Care

Gavril Hercz, M.D., F.R.C.P.C.
Associate Professor, Department of Medicine, University
of Toronto; Acting Director, Division of Nephrology, The
Wellesley Central Hospital, Toronto, Ontario, Canada

*System- and Problem-Oriented Evaluation (Renal
Manifestations)*

Mary Anne Huggins, M.D.C.M., C.C.F.P.
Director, Palliative Medicine, Toronto Hospital, General
Division, Toronto, Ontario, Canada

Palliative Care and Pain Management

Gabor Kandel, M.D., F.R.C.P.C.
Assistant Professor, University of Toronto, Faculty of
Medicine, University of Toronto; The Wellesley Central
Hospital, Toronto, Ontario, Canada

*System- and Problem-Oriented Evaluation
(Gastrointestinal Manifestations)*

George J. Kasupski, Ph.D., R.M.(C.C.M.)
Assistant Professor, University of Toronto; Senior
Scientist, Microbix Biosystems, Toronto, Ontario, Canada
*HIV Primary Care Evaluation and Management
(HIV Tests)*

Susan M. King, M.D., C.M.
Associate Professor of Paediatrics, University of Toronto;
Assistant Director of HIV/AIDS Program and Associate
Professor of Paediatrics, Division of Infectious Diseases,
The Hospital for Sick Children, Toronto, Ontario, Canada
Pediatric HIV

Ronald MacDonald, M.D., F.R.C.P.C.
Division of Neurology, Department of Medicine, The
Wellesley Central Hospital, Toronto, Ontario, Canada
*System- and Problem-Oriented Evaluation (Central
Nervous System Manifestations)*

Carol J. Major, B.Sc., M.L.T.
Head, HIV Laboratory, Central Public Health Laboratory,
Ontario Ministry of Health, Toronto, Ontario, Canada
*HIV Primary Care Evaluation and Management
(HIV Tests)*

Maggie Jane Marchand, B.Sc.
Clinical Dietitian—HIV Program, Registered Dietitian,
The Wellesley Central Hospital, Toronto, Ontario, Canada
System- and Problem-Oriented Evaluation (Nutrition)

Krystyna Ostrowska, M.D., F.R.C.P.C.
Medical Microbiologist, Infectious Diseases Specialist,
The Mississauga Hospital, Mississauga, Ontario, Canada
*System- and Problem-Oriented Evaluation (Central
Nervous System Manifestations), (Cryptococcal
Meningitis), (Toxoplasmosis)*

R. Scott Rowand
Assistant Professor, Departments of Health Administration
and Family and Community Medicine, University of
Toronto; President and CEO, The Wellesley Central
Hospital, Toronto, Ontario, Canada
*The Organization and Integration of Services for
Individuals with HIV*

Jane Sanders, R.N.
Clinical Co-ordinator, General Medicine, The Wellesley
Central Hospital, Toronto, Ontario, Canada
*Psychiatric and Psychosocial Issues (HIV Team
Approach)*

Carol Sawka, M.D., F.R.C.P.C.
Assistant Professor, Faculty of Medicine, University of Toronto; Division of Medical Oncology/Hematology, Toronto–Sunnybrook Regional Cancer Centre, Toronto, Ontario, Canada

System- and Problem-Oriented Evaluation (Oncologic Manifestations)

Susan Shurtleff, R.N., C.I.C.
Instructor, Centennial College of Applied Arts and Technology, Scarborough; Coordinator, Infection Control, The Wellesley Central Hospital, Toronto, Ontario, Canada

HIV Primary Care Evaluation and Management (Occupational Exposure); System- and Problem-Oriented Evaluation (Tuberculosis)

Dalia Slonim, Psy.D., C.Psych.
Adjunct–Internship supervisor, York University, Northern York; Psychologist, The Wellesley Central Hospital, Toronto, Ontario, Canada

Psychiatric and Psychosocial Issues (Psychotherapy with Individuals Suffering From a Devastating Illness)

The Rev. Peter Thompson, B.A., M.Div.
Order of Ministry: United Church of Canada, Toronto South Presbytery; Chaplain: The Wellesley Central Hospital; Specialist, Institutional Ministry: Canadian Association for Pastoral Education and Practice; The Wellesley Central Hospital, The United Church of Canada, Toronto South Presbytery, Toronto, Ontario, Canada

Psychiatric and Psychosocial Issues (Spirituality), (Care for the Care Giver)

Alice Tseng, Pharm.D.
Lecturer, Faculty of Pharmacy, University of Toronto; Immunodeficiency Clinic Pharmacist, The Toronto Hospital, Toronto, Ontario, Canada

System- and Problem-Oriented Evaluation (Cytomegalovirus), (Adverse Drug Reactions in HIV Patients), (Drug Interactions in HIV Patients); Adverse Effects of HIV Drugs: Incidence and Management; Drug Desensitization Protocols; Drug–Drug Interactions; Drug–Food Interactions

Ken Uffen, M.D., C.C.F.P.

Assistant Professor, University of Toronto, Faculty of Medicine; Residency Program Director, Department of Family and Community Medicine, North York General Hospital, Toronto, Ontario, Canada

HIV Primary Care Evaluation and Management (Medical Evaluation and Management)

Georgina Veldhorst, R.N., M.Sc.

Program Manager, The Wellesley Central Hospital, Toronto, Ontario, Canada

An Approach to Patients with HIV (Partnering in Care); The Role of Nursing in HIV/AIDS Care

Sharon Walmsley, M.D., F.R.C.P.C.

Assistant Professor, Departments of Medicine and Microbiology, University of Toronto, Assistant Director Immunodeficiency Clinic, Division of Infectious Diseases, The Toronto Hospital, Toronto, Ontario, Canada

Women and HIV

Peter A. Williams

Volunteer Team Leader, HIV Program, The Wellesley Central Hospital; Community and Volunteer Educator, Casey House Hospice, Inc., Community Programs, Toronto, Ontario, Canada

An Approach to Patients with HIV (The Role of Advocacy in Patient Care)

Tong Yeung, M.D., B.B.S., M.R.C.P.(UK), F.C.C.P.

Clinical Fellow, Department of Medicine, Toronto Hospital, General Division, Toronto, Ontario, Canada

System- and Problem-Oriented Evaluation (Cytomegalovirus) (Herpes Simplex Virus), (Varicella-Zoster Virus)

PREFACE

This manual was inspired by concerns expressed by members of the HIV community who were working with the Wellesley Hospital in Toronto, Canada, to improve the care of HIV patients. As a teaching hospital there was continual turnover of the medical caregivers and an urgent need to provide simple and practical guidelines for the evaluation and treatment of HIV infection and its complications. A committee contributed to the development of the framework for the manual and a first edition was piloted locally. Following extensive feedback from caregivers in the inpatient, outpatient, and emergency settings who used the manual for several months, revisions were made and new sections were added to produce the current edition.

The manual targets all members of the team caring for individuals with HIV. The chapters are intended to be brief and provide a practical overview with specific recommendations where appropriate. Key references are provided at the end of each chapter for further reading.

ACKNOWLEDGMENTS

Several individuals contributed to the development of this manual. Members of the committee were: Dr. C. Chan, Anne Conlin, Dr. B. Cornelson, Dr. M. Fanning, Dr. G. Kandel, Ms. J. Lee, Ms. M. J. Marchand, Dr. K. Ostrowska, Dr. K. Uffen, Mr. R. Van Dusen, Dr. T. Yeung. Anne Conlin coordinated the committee process, collated contributors' materials and directed the final production of the manuscript. Mary O'Callahan provided secretarial support to the committee and to the contributors, producing the final manuscript.

CONTENTS

Color Plates Follow

COLOR PLATES

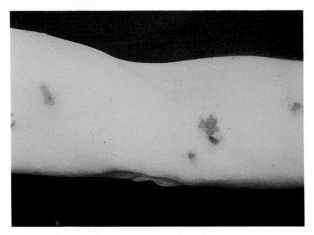

Kaposi's Sarcoma

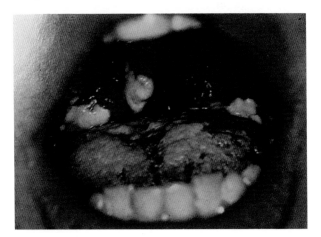

Oral thrush

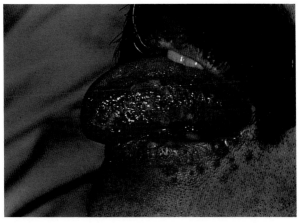

Oral hairy leupoplakia and Peri-oral Herpes simplex

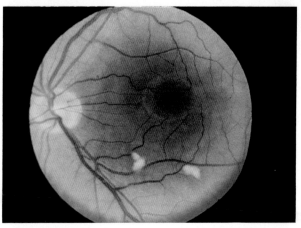

Cotton-wool spots, retina

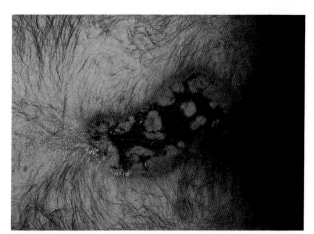

Peri-anal Herpes simplex (HSV-2) infection

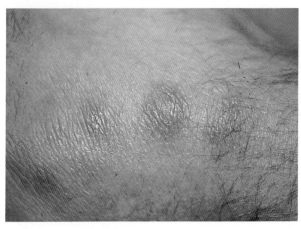

Bacillary Angiomatosis

Introduction to HIV

Mary Fanning, M.D., Ph.D., F.R.C.P.C., F.A.C.P.

Acquired immune deficiency syndrome (AIDS) is a clinical syndrome that involves progressive immune deficiency and consequent development of opportunistic infections, tumors, neurologic disease, and systemic wasting. The underlying immune deficiency is caused by infection with human immunodeficiency virus type 1 (HIV-1), which can be contracted through sexual activity, from receipt of infected blood or blood products, or transplacentally.

Once inside the bloodstream, the virus enters host cells by attaching to the CD4 cell membrane antigen, which serves as its receptor for cell entry. Inside the CD4 cell, the virus transcribes itself into DNA using the enzyme reverse transcriptase, integrates into the host DNA, and produces more virus, leading to increased viral load and infection of more CD4 cells. The majority of CD4 cells are lymphocytes, but macrophages, monocytes, and a variety of cells from other tissues, such as skin, gastrointestinal tract, or central nervous system, also have CD4 receptors and can be directly infected by HIV.

Acute HIV infection can cause a mononucleosis-like syndrome that is self-resolving. Early on during HIV infection, the virus may go into an apparent clinically latent period and the immune system continues to function relatively normally. However, the virus is actively replicating in the lymph nodes and immune dysregulation, particularly of the B-cell system, and lymphokine activation may occur, producing a rise in immunoglobulins and a decrease in the ability to mount an antibody response to new antigens or immunizations/vaccines. During this period, infected individuals may remain asymptomatic or show persistent generalized lymphadenopathy. Some may develop thrombocytopenia as a result of immunologic factors.

As the disease progresses, but before an "AIDS indicator" condition is diagnosed, individuals may experience various symptoms, such as unexplained fever, night sweats, weight loss, fatigue, and diarrhea. The cell-mediated immune system is progressively impaired by viral replication, leading to dysfunction and ultimately to serious depletion of CD4 lymphocytes. When the absolute CD4 cell count falls to between 200 and 400, HIV-positive patients may experience minor opportunistic infections, such as candidiasis (thrush), herpes-zoster (shingles), tinea pedis (athlete's foot), and oral hairy leukoplakia. Chronic skin conditions, such as seborrheic dermatitis, may also flare up.

With further impairment of the immune system, more severe opportunistic infections, such as *Pneumocystis carinii* pneumonia, may appear, but usually only when the CD4 count falls to <200, and some, such as cytomegalovirus (CMV) or *mycobacterium avium* complex (MAC), occur primarily with CD4 counts <50.

Tumors, such as Kaposi's sarcoma or lymphoma, central nervous system disease, and severe wasting are additional indicators of progression to AIDS.

A recently proposed expansion of the surveillance case definition for AIDS classifies patients according to their clinical condition and CD4 count. Clinical conditions are classified as (A) asymptomatic, (B) symptomatic, and (C) AIDS-indicator conditions.

In group B, several conditions have recently been added, including recurrent bacterial pneumonia and vulvovaginal candidiasis. AIDS-indicator conditions now include cervical cancer and tuberculosis in addition to tumors and opportunistic infections. CD4 counts are classified as category 1, ≥500; category 2, 200 to 499; and category 3, <200.

In general, therapeutic approaches to this infection attempt to maintain a good immunologic status by controlling viral replication with antiretroviral agents, preventive therapy against opportunistic infections, and aggressive investigation and treatment of opportunistic infections when they occur.

Suggested Reading

1. 1993 Revised classification system for HIV infection and expanded surveillance case definition for AIDS among adolescents and adults. MMWR 1993; 41(RR17): 1–19.

An Approach to Patients with HIV

▬ SUGGESTED APPROACH TO PATIENTS WITH HIV

Mary Fanning, M.D., Ph.D., F.R.C.P.C., F.A.C.P.

HIV infection denotes a catastrophic illness affecting primarily young people in the prime of life. A diagnosis of HIV infection therefore has a devastating impact, even if the person seems perfectly healthy when given the diagnosis. The psychological implications may be particularly searing, as the infected person contemplates a downward path and future losses. In adjusting to their illness, patients with HIV infection experience many emotions, particularly anxiety, depression, and anger. Physicians and other health care professionals must be prepared to show understanding and accept the anger that may be directed at both the doctor and the health care system. An empathetic approach, compassion, and patience in dealing with the medical complexities of AIDS are crucial for physicians and other health care professionals who wish to earn the confidence of their patients.

Many of those diagnosed with HIV are well informed about their disease and may in fact know a good deal more than their doctors. They will often want to be in control of and share in their therapy. Physicians and the HIV team should be willing to discuss new treatments and learn about them from their patients. If the new information is incorporated into the current approach to treatment, physician and patient can jointly explore information about any new therapy proposed. This partnership gives the patient a sense of autonomy while also providing the support and wisdom of medical expertise. Patients may understandably be distressed if they feel their physician does not know anything about HIV treatment when in fact the doctor is simply not conversant with one particular treatment or a new therapy. Those with HIV need to have trust and confidence in their care givers and should feel that their doctor has an open mind to new therapeutic approaches.

As the HIV epidemic spreads, it is affecting people with more diverse cultural and social backgrounds. There is still a great stigma attached to an HIV-positive test result, which adds to the problems those affected must face. People with HIV often find questions about their sexual behavior and the way they acquired HIV inappropriate and upsetting when they are seeking medical advice because of serious symptoms such as fever or shortness of breath. However, in some cases, questions about IV drug use, sexual activities, or use of blood components may be pertinent to their illness and its treatment.

When evaluating a person with HIV infection, physicians should keep in mind that these patients may also experience disease processes not associated with HIV, but consistent with their age and medical background. In addition, symptoms linked to HIV may be subtle and subclinical.

■ PARTNERING IN CARE
Georgina Veldhorst, R.N., M.Sc.

Limited attention has been given to the importance of the development of a partnership between the patient and the care provider to patient outcomes and satisfaction. Traditionally, the reality in health care has been one in which the patients serve the care providers. When patients enter the hospital, they are informed that they must wear hospital gowns, fit into hospital routines, take medications at prescribed times, and have visitors during specified times, and are requested to comply with many other institutional routines and rituals. Over the last decade a number of new approaches to the patient–health care system relationship have been attempted. Some of these include care providers using customer-oriented approaches, whereby organizational structures are changed into programs, services, or clusters according to patient need. All of these systems have some merit and shortcomings. No system or organizational structure can be effective if the care providers do not enter into a partnership with the patient and his or her family or loved ones.

A partnership can be defined as a relationship in which two or more people have a joint interest.[1] In health care, a partnership between care provider and patient is a relationship that values and integrates that patient's perspective with the knowledge and expertise of the care provider.

In a study conducted by Gerteis and co-workers,[2] seven dimensions that patients considered important in their care were identified. These dimensions will be presented as they relate to patients with HIV/AIDS entering into a patient–care provider relationship.

RESPECT FOR VALUES, PREFERENCES, AND EXPRESSED NEEDS

Respect for values entails respecting the patient's lifestyle, cultural values, religious beliefs, and chosen significant others. Respecting preferences includes respecting the patient's choice with regard to HIV status disclosure and maintaining confidentiality with all others. Maintaining this confidentiality may mean integrating HIV services with other services so that visitors cannot draw conclusions about a patient's diagnosis. In order to enter the partnership, the care provider must determine the long- and short-term goals of the patient, the patient's meaning of "quality of life," and the patient's expectations of the partnership with the care provider(s).

The provider has a responsibility to determine the extent of the patient's desire to be involved in decision making. This involvement may change over time. Some individuals may want to have full control and view care providers as consultants. Other patients may want their care providers to take more control.

After the initial diagnosis of HIV is made, it is generally not necessary for care providers to know how the patient contracted the virus. Regardless of how the patient contracted HIV, the patient and his or her significant others should be treated with sensitivity, dignity, and respect.

COORDINATION AND INTEGRATION OF CARE

Patients are concerned about who is in charge and who coordinates their care. Patients with HIV generally use the health care system many times over the course of their illness. Do they see the same care providers each time? Do the care providers communicate with each other? Is there communication and coordination between primary care physicians, inpatient physicians, nurses, and other interdisciplinary team members? A system of continuity of care givers and continuity in care may decrease the patient's feeling of vulnerability.

INFORMATION, COMMUNICATION, AND EDUCATION

Information about HIV/AIDS is changing rapidly. Whereas traditionally, care providers have been most knowledgable about treatments, they may encounter patients who are more informed about HIV/AIDS management than some of their care providers. Some patients maintain a record of their own test results. They may have questions about or use complementary therapies. Although some feel threatened by knowledgeable, and thus empowered patients, the role of the care provider is to enable patients to meet their own goals regarding the management of their own care.

PHYSICAL COMFORT

Many patients are concerned about the pain and suffering associated with HIV/AIDS. Pain management is a large component of living with HIV/AIDS. Do care providers listen to patient complaints and act upon them? As patients become increasingly ill with this disease, they require much greater assistance with activities of daily living. Are their needs for privacy and dignity maintained? Have their physical surroundings been altered so as to prevent falls and other injuries? Do care providers consider the needs of patients with regard to visiting hours? Some patients may want someone to stay with them at night.

EMOTIONAL SUPPORT AND ALLEVIATION OF FEAR AND ANXIETY

Patients with HIV/AIDS may have anxiety about maintaining confidentiality about their HIV status. They may fear losing their jobs or their health insurance, or abandonment by family and friends. Patients may worry about maintaining their independence or the impact of their illness on their partner or family. As many HIV/AIDS patients are no longer able to work, may not have life insurance or adequate health care insurance, and require costly treatments, financial issues are often a great concern. If other family members (partner, spouse, or child) are also infected, caring for family members or dying before their child may be a source of anxiety.

INVOLVEMENT OF FAMILY AND FRIENDS

In caring for patients with HIV/AIDS, it is very important to determine from patients who they want involved in their care. Significant others may not be traditional family members, and their selection should be respected by the providers. The patient's partner, spouse, or child may also be infected and may also need support. Care providers should also be ready to support the patient and his or her family if the patient wishes to disclose the diagnosis. This can be very stressful for both the patient and family.

TRANSITION AND CONTINUITY

A smooth transition from the hospital or clinic to the community and back to the hospital is very important, as is continuity in care, regardless of the point of service. Continuity of care givers from one visit to the hospital to the next may lessen the patient's stress.

In summary, partnering with patients and their loved ones begins with the individual care provider. The seven dimensions can be used as a guide to get to know a patient's "story." A thorough understanding of this dynamic story facilitates appropriate decision making by the care provider. When the care provider partners with the patient and those closest to the patient by addressing and integrating these seven dimensions into the care, the patient is likely to experience much less frustration, and the care provider more likely to encounter a patient who is content with the care being given.

References

1. Brown L (Ed). The New Shorter Oxford English Dictionary, 5th Edition, Vol. II, p. 2111. Oxford: Clarendon Press, 1993.
2. Gerteis M, Edgman-Levitan S, Daley J. Introduction: Medicine and Health from the Patient's Perspective. In Gerteis M, Edgman-Levitan S, Daley J (Eds), Through the Patient's Eyes: Understanding and Promoting Patient Centered Care, pp. 1–15. San Francisco: Jossey-Bass Publishers, 1993.

■ THE ROLE OF ADVOCACY IN PATIENT CARE

Mary Fanning, M.D., Ph.D., F.R.C.P.C., F.A.C.P.
Peter Williams

Trends in medical care are slowly shifting the emphasis to client-centered decision making. In the care of HIV-positive individuals, this trend has been accelerated and represents a new challenge to health care professionals not accustomed to this approach. In addition, HIV patients frequently seek the involvement of a variety of people who represent relationships of significance in their lives. Coordinating care and decision making in this context requires new approaches, respect for the wishes of the patient, flexibility, and careful attention to communication.

In the medical setting, care of the patient with HIV involves a team of health care professionals. In addition, a volunteer team and a patient- or family-selected lay care team may be involved with the patient's medical care and comfort. These lay individuals should be involved in all "team" meetings. The appointment of an advocate selected by the patient from this group will facilitate the discussion of issues and decision making. This extended team should be encouraged to define terms (e.g., palliative care) in order to promote a common understanding, to clarify who should be present at "family meetings" and who will be the spokesperson, and to discuss differences between the wishes of the patient and those of "family or friends."

To enhance the role of the advocate, health care professionals need to be prepared to relinquish some control in decision making to the patient or advocate and establish a common understanding of issues. One must first listen and then seek to understand the advocate's position and the patient's wishes without becoming defensive. Clear and specific guidelines about when to call the physician will diminish anxiety. Encouraging the patient and care team to keep a logbook at home can help to objectify the situation. Discussing potential situations ("What happens if . . . ") can avert a crisis.

Physicians caring for patients in the community may come to feel isolated. Connecting with a medical or lay care team can enhance the resources available to the patient. Health care professionals should be sensitive to the fears of patients surrounding their medical visits. Institutions should support their staff by providing training to deal with advocacy and encouraging involvement in the community and awareness of the information the patient is receiving in the community.

Patient and advocate paticipation in medical decision making can greatly increase the satisfaction with care for this chronic terminal illness.

HIV Primary Care Evaluation and Management

HIV TESTING

Brian Cornelson, M.D., C.C.F.P.

As discussed in Chapter 2, a diagnosis of HIV infection carries profound and far-reaching implications for a person's health and well-being. It is therefore essential that anyone tested be properly assessed and prepared for such a diagnosis and assured the availability of the necessary support and follow-up care. The physician who orders an HIV test must ensure that these conditions are met. Expectation of a negative result by either the patient or the physician does *not* relieve the physician of this responsibility. Unexpected positive results are not uncommon, and being able to respond to them appropriately and effectively is possibly the greatest challenge that physicians face in ordering HIV tests.

Generally speaking, a hospital inpatient ward is not the ideal site for HIV testing because

- many hospital stays are shorter than the time lapse between initiating testing and obtaining a result; therefore,

- most patients will no longer be available in hospital for the appropriate post-test counseling, and

- it is impossible to guarantee patients the high degree of confidentiality that HIV testing requires. In addition,

- in most situations, acute management must be instituted on the basis of clinical presentation before the result of the test will be available.

Therefore, it is rarely in the patient's best interest to initiate HIV testing in hospital. The only indications for HIV testing in a hospitalized patient are

- the presence of an illness *possibly* related to HIV infection where management would be materially different if the person were *known* to be HIV-infected; and

- after a health care worker has sustained significant exposure to a patient's blood or bodily fluids, and the patient's HIV status is unknown.

Apart from these specific situations, it may also be appropriate to offer or suggest HIV testing to certain patients in ambulatory clinics, provided appropriate pre- and post-test counseling and guarantees of confidentiality are given. Testing may also be done on patients in family practice teaching units, where attending physicians are the patients' primary care givers. It is *never* appropriate to initiate HIV testing in the Emergency Department, as the result will not be available in time to affect a management decision.

In those selected situations where it *is* appropriate to initiate HIV testing of hospitalized patients, the following guidelines help to ensure that this procedure meets the medical and emotional needs of the person being tested. The principles and procedures outlined below are also suitable for family practice teaching units, physicians' offices, and other ambulatory settings.

PRINCIPLES

1. HIV testing must be done only when appropriate pre-test and post-test counseling is assured. The procedures for counseling are outlined below.

2. Pre-test counseling must be done by an appropriately trained physician (attending physician, consultant, or house staff) or other health care worker who conducts a thorough and sensitive pre-test assessment, using an approved HIV pre-test protocol.

3. The health care worker conducting the test should also take this opportunity to provide appropriate patient education. People are far more receptive to information about risk reduction *before* being tested than at the post-test visit, when they tend to hear little other than the result itself because of their primary feelings of relief if the result is negative.

4. Arrangements for post-test counseling should be made by the health care worker who does the pre-test counseling. A staff or consulting physician may give the result to the patient at his or her office. If a member of

the house staff does the pre-test counseling, he or she must ensure that the result will be forwarded to and given by the attending physician if the house staff will not be immediately available when the result arrives.

Health care workers doing the post-test counseling should use their institution's HIV post-test protocol. They must be able to give and explain the significance of negative, indeterminate, and positive results, and provide the necessary immediate support and follow-up recommendations to someone with an indeterminate or positive result.

5. The laboratory will not process a request for HIV testing unless it is accompanied by a properly completed *HIV serology* requisition form *and* an accompanying *HIV test requisition* form, which should contain the following:

   ▪ A signed request for HIV testing from the patient's attending physician, if other than the person doing the pre- and post-test counseling (e.g., a house staff or consultant physician or other health care worker).

   ▪ A signed declaration by the person who has done the pre-test counseling, stating that
     —the patient has been given the necessary pre-test counseling;
     —appropriate arrangements have been made to provide post-test counseling along with the test result;
     —the patient has signed an informed *HIV test consent form,* which has been placed on the chart; and
     —the patient has agreed to return in person at a specified time and place to obtain the result.

6. If a request for HIV testing is initiated by the *patient,* he or she should normally be referred to his or her family physician or to an anonymous testing facility (see 9, below).

7. If a request for HIV testing is initiated by a physician *other than* the patient's primary physician, he or she must explain the reason for this request, specifically, the *medical* indications for testing. Knowledge or presumption of a patient's past or present risk activity alone is *not* an indication for suggesting an HIV test. These situations may, however, be an appropriate reason for the person's primary care or family physician to raise the issue of HIV testing. Patients who require HIV testing (for the purposes of organ transplants, for example) must also be given pre- and post-test counseling. As with any

test situation, the health care worker who will be providing the result must be prepared to help the person deal with an unexpected positive result.

8. A health care provider may initiate a request that a patient be tested for HIV if the provider has sustained a needle-stick injury or other serious exposure to a patient's blood or bodily fluids. The procedure in this situation is detailed in the hospital's AIDS staff-related issues policy. In this situation, patients must again be given appropriate pre- and post-test counseling, according to these protocols, by an occupational health nurse. *In addition,* they must give written consent to the provision of their test result to the occupational health nurse, who will notify the health care provider that the person to whose bodily fluids they were exposed is or is not HIV positive. *A patient cannot be compelled to undergo testing, regardless of the circumstances.*

9. The health care worker must explain the availability of *anonymous* testing, which is done at specifically designated sites, and *nominal* or *non-nominal* (coded) testing, which can be done in hospitals, laboratories, and doctors' offices. In anonymous testing, there are no patient-specific identifiers on the requisition. The only way to connect an individual with a result is through the numeric identifier given to the person being tested. In nominal testing, the individual's name is used. In non-nominal testing, a code is used. This *increases confidentiality* but is not *anonymous,* because there must be a way for the *person doing the test* to connect an individual to a test result. People must be told that they have had an HIV test and its result will become part of their medical records if they are tested at the hospital or through their physician's office. Nominal testing is strongly encouraged when HIV testing is done at the request of a health care provider following accidental exposure.

10. In order to proceed with testing, health care workers must be familiar with the pre- and post-test protocols, which follow.

HIV PRE-TEST PROTOCOL
Preamble

Pre-test counseling must be done in complete privacy to promote confidence and openness in the person being tested.

If counseling is done in an inpatient setting, it must *not* be conducted on the ward, where the conversation may be overheard by others.

People being tested for HIV often experience considerable anxiety and apprehension. The person may fear criticism or judgment for engaging in risk activities linked to HIV infection, and may deny such activities if he or she perceives the health care worker who does the test to be insensitive or moralistic. Some patients will feel more comfortable if they already know and have a good relationship with the health care worker who gives the counseling, hence the advantage of this being done by the primary care physician. Others will prefer the anonymity of being tested by someone *not* known.

Preparation

The health care worker doing pre-test counseling should be knowledgeable about and able to explain the following:

- the basic facts about acute HIV infection, transmission, and the immune response to HIV infection;
- the long-term effects of HIV infection;
- the difference between HIV infection and AIDS;
- known HIV risk activities and characteristics;
- essential facts about HIV testing, including
  —the test(s) that will be used;
  —the incidence and causes of false-positive and false-negative results;
  —recommended follow-up for those with a positive result.

The health care worker should also feel comfortable about discussing HIV risk activities, be at ease, and be able to appear nonjudgmental and supportive, regardless of his or her personal beliefs and values.

The health care worker doing pre-test counseling should have ready the following documents:

- The hospital HIV pre-test protocol (this document).
- The hospital HIV test consent (Fig. 3–1).
- The hospital HIV test requisition (Fig. 3–2).
- The HIV serology requisition (see Fig. 3–3).

The counseling should be done in a place where the conversation cannot be overheard and where it can be done without interruption (by phone calls, pagers, etc.).

1. I, _____ , a patient at _____ ,
   agree to have an HIV antibody test. HIV is the virus
   linked to AIDS (acquired immune deficiency syndrome).

2. I understand the following:

   - a *positive* HIV test does not by itself mean that I have
     AIDS;

   - a *negative* HIV test does not necessarily mean that I am
     NOT infected by HIV.

   - I can be tested *anonymously* for HIV elsewhere.

   - this test result will be part of my permanent medical
     record at _____ .

3. I agree that

   - I have had pre-test counseling for this test;

   - I understand the meaning of this test and its possible
     results; and

   - I have given the person who conducted the pre-test
     counseling correct information.

4. I agree that I will receive my HIV test result in person and
   that I will participate in the necessary post-test counseling.

5. I will obtain my test result from

   Dr. _____ at _____

   (Location)

   Signed: _____ Date: _____

   Witness: _____

■■■■■■ FIGURE 3-1
HIV Test Consent

Procedure

Health care workers should do the following as part of the
HIV pre-test counseling session:

1. Ensure that the patient knows that the purpose of the test
   is to detect the presence of *antibody* to the virus that is
   associated with AIDS.

2. Explain *why* the test is being done:
   —because the person has a medical condition that could
   be related to HIV infection;

1. I, _____ , the attending physician of the patient named in the HIV test consent, request that an HIV test be performed on this patient.

   Signed: _____   Date: _____

2. I, _____ , attending physician ____ / consultant physician ____ /house staff physician ____ / (other: specify) _____ ,

   - have provided the appropriate HIV pre-test counseling to this patient, following the HIV pre-test protocol;
   - have completed the virology HIV serology requisition form correctly to the best of my knowledge;
   - have obtained the patient's written informed consent for HIV testing, which is on the patient's chart; and
   - have provided the patient with information he or she needs to obtain the result of this test.

   Signed: _____   Date: _____

■■■■■■   FIGURE 3-2
HIV Test Requisition

   —because the person is a prospective donor (of organs, semen, etc.);
   —because the person has requested the test;
   —because a health care worker has had a significant (i.e., potentially infectious) exposure to the patient's bodily fluids;
   —other (specify).

3. Ensure that the patient is aware
   —that the test is *not* a test for AIDS, but that it is a test for the presence of antibodies to the human immunodeficiency virus (HIV), which indicates probable infection with HIV;
   —that the test result will be part of his or her medical record;
   —that anonymous testing is available at other sites;
   —that he or she must come in person to obtain the test result and appropriate post-test counseling.

4. Fill in the address section of the HIV serology requisi-

Ministry of Health Ontario	Laboratory Services Branch	VIROLOGY HIV 1/2 SEROLOGY	**PHL USE ONLY**	
			Date Rec'd	PHL No.

Patient Identification	Previous HIV Serology PHL No. or anonymous test code

Date of Birth yy / mm / dd	Sex: ☐ M ☐ F	Date Specimen Collected yy / mm / dd	Doctor's (area code) Phone No.
☐ VISA Requirement		Sender's Reference No. 1 3 ⫶ 0 9 5	

Please print/stamp doctor's name and address clearly and firmly on all copies. Include postal Code. Provide one address only, in the unshaded area.

```
THE WELLESLEY HOSPITAL
WELLESLEY HEALTH CENTRE
410 SHERBOURNE ST.
TORONTO, ONT.
M4X 1K2        D-78-1
```

CONFIDENTIAL WHEN COMPLETED

PATIENT'S SYMPTOMS/DIAGNOSIS

☐ None
☐ Fever
☐ Fatigue
☐ Diarrhea
☐ Skin Rash
☐ Weight Loss
☐ Night Sweats

☐ Decreased helper cell number
☐ Recurrent oral candidiasis
☐ Kaposi's Sarcoma
☐ Generalized Lymphadenopathy
☐ PCP
☐ ARC/Pre-AIDS
☐ AIDS

Other (Specify) _____

Date of Onset

PATIENT RISK (Check all applicable boxes)

☑ has had sex with men
☑ has had sex with women
☐ needle use
☐ sex partner of HIV + person
☐ sex partner of person(s) at risk for HIV
☐ Other (Specify) _____

☐ recipient of blood products before 1/11/85
☐ recipient of blood transfusion before 1/11/85
☐ endemic area immigrant / traveller
☐ offspring of HIV + mother
☐ no identifiable risk

PHL USE ONLY

SCREENING TEST (ELISA)

CONFIRMATORY TEST

☐ Supplemental (ELISA)

☐ Immunoblot

REMARKS

☐ No ID on sample tube
☐ Further report to follow

Date Reported _____

1210-44 (94/04)   (see over for information)

FIGURE 3–3

Virology, HIV Serology Requisition Form Used at the Wellesley Hospital, Toronto. *Ontario Ministry of Health, HIV Laboratory, reprinted by permission.*

tion form, indicating the name of the *attending* or *consultant physician* who will receive the report.

5. Complete the *Patient's Symptoms/Diagnosis* and *Patient Risk* sections of the HIV serology requisition form. In order to get the necessary information, health care workers must be sensitive, open-minded and nonjudgmental, doing their best to make the patient comfortable and willing to disclose all possible risk activities. The

interview may require the health care worker to explain things about which both he or she and the patient may be unfamiliar or uncomfortable. Being frank and straightforward helps to minimize the discomfort, reduce the tension, and engender a trusting atmosphere.

Neutral questions minimize potential embarrassment and promote full disclosure. For example, start with the question, "Are you currently or have you ever been sexually active?" If the answer is affirmative, ask, "Are you sexually active with men or women or both?" This gets around assuming someone's sexual orientation—or forcing the person to label him or herself. (Many men sometimes have sex with other men but do not identify themselves as being homosexual.) Then ask, "Do you have a regular partner, casual partners, or both?" Ask if the patient has ever had unprotected sex; if so, how recently, what type(s), and with roughly how many different partners over his or her lifetime. This will allow you to roughly gauge the risk of exposure to the virus.

Accurate completion of the HIV serology requisition will allow laboratory staff to handle the specimen appropriately, including the use of tests in addition to the enzyme-linked immunosorbent assay (ELISA) if indicated on the basis of symptoms or risks, even if the initial ELISA is negative.

6. Ask the person for the date of the most recent known risk activity for HIV infection. If it has been within the past 14 weeks, explain that a negative result may not necessarily mean the absence of recent HIV infection. It can take 14 weeks, and occasionally longer, for an infected person to seroconvert. Therefore, a test done in this "window period" may not be accurate, and the person may prefer to wait for the test until at least 14 weeks have elapsed since the last known high-risk exposure or activity. If the exposure has a greater-than-expected probability of being infectious (e.g., unprotected receptive sex or shared needle use with a known HIV-positive person), a second test 6 months after the exposure is warranted if the first test is negative.

7. Explain the test procedure:

- If the initial ELISA screening test is *negative,* no further testing is necessary;

- If the ELISA is *positive,* a Western blot confirmatory test will be done on the same sample of blood.

Potential Western blot results include the following:

- *Negative* result: probable false-positive ELISA or possible early seroconversion. If the test was done in the window period, it must be repeated in 3 months.

- *Positive* result: highly probable HIV infection.*

- *Indeterminate* result: inconclusive, must be repeated in 3 months. If still indeterminate in 3 months, HIV infection is unlikely. Will usually require referral to an infectious disease consultant.

8. Explain that it will take 2 to 3 weeks to obtain the test result. Generally, a negative ELISA result will be available earlier than a positive one, in which case the test will be repeated and the confirmatory Western blot done.

9. Ask the patient whether he or she expects the test to be positive or negative. If a negative result is expected, but you consider a positive result possible, based on information from the patient or on his or her medical condition, explain briefly but clearly that you think there is some possibility that the result *may* be positive, giving the reasons for your concern, in order to help the person prepare for a positive result.

10. If the person asks what you think the result will be, try to be honest and *not* provide any false reassurances, regardless of what *you* expect (the patient may have withheld some information). It is reasonable to say, "I cannot predict your result, but based on the information you have given me, I think it is (either/or) unlikely/possible that your test may be positive." A false reassurance will only make more difficult giving the person who is expecting a negative test a positive result.

False-positive/false-negative results: False-negative results most commonly occur because the test was done in the window between the time of infection and the development of antibody to the virus. The sensitivity of the ELISA is at least 99.5 percent, and the specificity is higher than 99.8 percent *in high-risk populations.* False-positive results can occur in the presence of autoreactive antibodies, severe hepatic disease, and passive immunoglobulin injections, after flu shots, and with some malignancies. When the ELISA and Western blot are done properly and used in combination, the predictive value of both being positive is well over 99 percent in persons at risk for HIV infection. However, this does *not* exclude the possibility of rare false-positive results, especially in low-risk individuals, confounded by the fact that not everyone will admit to engaging in risk activities.

11. Ask the patient how he or she would react if the test result came back positive. Some people are unsure, and may elect to postpone testing until they have had time to think about it.

12. Ask the person what support systems (spouse/partner/ lover, family, friends, etc.) he or she can turn to should the test result be positive.

13. Ask if the person has a family physician familiar with the management of HIV. If not, or if the patient doesn't know, inform the patient that you will provide the name of an HIV primary care physician, if requested or desired. No one should engage in HIV pre-test counseling without being able to provide such an assurance.

14. Ask whether everything you have said has been well understood and if the person has any questions, and answer them.

15. Ask whether the person still wishes to go ahead with the HIV test. If yes, complete the HIV test consent form. Review the statements (which cover things you have already explained) and ask him or her to sign the consent in the appropriate place. File the test consent in the patient's chart.

16. Explain that blood will be drawn for the HIV test, and that the result will arrive in about 3 weeks. Give the patient written instructions telling him or her where to go for the test result and who will provide it, if it will be someone other than yourself.

17. Complete the hospital HIV test requisition form, staple it to the HIV serology requisition form, and hand it in to the nursing station or send it with the patient to the laboratory.

HIV POST-TEST PROTOCOL

As with pre-test counseling, it is essential to provide the HIV test result and post-test counseling in complete privacy.

Giving a Negative Result

1. If the ELISA is *negative,* tell the person that he or she *probably* does not have HIV infection. However, the result may not be accurate if he or she engaged in high-risk activities within the 14 weeks prior to testing. Occasionally it can take up to 6 months for a person who

has been infected to seroconvert. For this reason, it is best to review the patient's risk activities in the past 6 months, and recommend retesting in an additional 3 to 6 months if the patient has been engaging in recent high-risk activity.

2. In the rare instance when the ELISA is *positive* and the Western blot *indeterminate,* explain the significance of this result and the necessity for further testing (see the HIV pre-test protocol for further explanation). Living with an equivocal result can be as stressful in the short term as getting a positive result.

3. Reinforce HIV risk reduction/avoidance. For sexually active people, this includes a detailed discussion of ways to reduce risks during various types of sexual activity. For injection drug users, it means giving instructions on obtaining or properly cleaning and not sharing needles. For everyone at risk of HIV it means not donating blood, semen, or organs.

The health care worker doing the post-test counseling should be knowledgeable about and comfortable with describing ways of reducing the risk of HIV transmission for all types of sexual activity and injection drug use. Telling people *not* to engage in certain sexual activities or injection drug use is not effective and is probably not appropriate. If people want to change their behaviors, they will do so or seek advice when they are ready for it from someone they trust.

Giving a Positive Result

1. It is difficult to tell someone that the HIV test was positive, given the tremendous medical and psychological implications of such a result. This reinforces the importance and value of pre-test counseling, in particular, discussion about how the person would react to a positive result and raising this possibility if the person has engaged in high-risk behaviors.

   In giving the result, it is best to avoid "beating around the bush" or trying to soften the blow. People who have had an HIV test are interested in only one thing: the result. If a patient has had a positive test, it is best to say simply, "Your HIV test was positive. This means that you have been infected with HIV." Give the patient time to absorb the news. The person may say nothing right away, may have an emotional response, or may start asking questions. It is best to begin by answering the person's questions. The patient will ask about the things that are uppermost in the mind at that time, and therefore this is the information the patient is most ready to hear—and remember. After you have answered the patient's questions, tell him or her that there are some other things you want to discuss, and proceed with the issues that follow.

2. Explain the significance of the result. If the ELISA and Western blot are *positive,* tell the person that he or she has been infected with HIV. He or she does *not* have AIDS unless there are also co-existent AIDS-defining conditions.

3. Emphasize that the person is *infectious* to others, and strongly emphasize risk reduction/elimination, as discussed in No. 3 of Giving a Negative Result. It is equally important for the HIV-positive individual to reduce risks of transmitting the infection to others *and* to avoid being *re*-infected him- or herself.

4. Ask again what personal supports the person has (friends, spouse/partner, family, family physician, etc.). Has he or she discussed the fact that he or she was being tested for HIV with anyone? Will he or she be able to disclose the result to them? It is *not* essential for people to disclose their result to anyone right away, although they must take steps to ensure that they do not put close contacts at continued risk of infection.

5. Advise the patient *not* to make any immediate decisions about personal and work commitments, such as quitting work or ending a relationship. People need time to respond to the impact of discovering that they are HIV-positive.

6. Emphasize that HIV infection is a long-term condition with which people can live for many years after being initially infected. Prevention and treatment is available for some of the complications of HIV infection that enable people to live longer and better than they have in the past.

7. Outline the next steps that need to be taken, including a complete physical assessment, assessment of immune function and other investigations, and immunizations. This should be undertaken by a physician who is knowledgeable about HIV disease and who can provide ongoing care. The individual who already has a family physician (who may or may not be knowledgeable about HIV infection) may wish to discuss this with him or her.

Alternately, he or she may wish to be referred to a (new) physician who is knowledgeable in this area. If so, refer the patient to an HIV primary care physician. *A patient must never leave an HIV post-test counseling session without the names and phone numbers of physicians who are accepting new HIV patients.*

8. Although it is important to cover all these topics, remember that patients will probably *not* remember most of what you have told them at the post-test counseling session. It will be helpful to jot down the important points that you have covered. This is also why it is usually a good idea to suggest to people that they bring a friend with them when they come to get their result.

▬▬▬ HIV TESTS

George Kasupski, Ph.D., R.M. (C.C.M.)

Carol Major, B.Sc., M.L.T.

ENZYME-LINKED IMMUNOSORBENT ASSAY

Screening and confirmatory tests are done routinely when HIV antibody testing is requested, interpretation being based on both tests.

Serologic screening to detect HIV antibody is the most common way to demonstrate HIV infection. The test currently used to screen serum for antibodies to HIV is the enzyme-linked immunosorbent assay (ELISA). It uses a mixture of synthetic peptides and/or recombinant proteins to detect antibodies to certain envelope proteins of both HIV-1 and HIV-2. Recent experience with HIV subtype O (for *Other*) has shown that some recombinant and peptide antigens do not bind to the antibodies produced to significant variants. This depends on the region of the genome cloned or synthesized and the degree of variance present in that part of the genome in the subtype. All HIV testing kits licensed for use in Canada should detect currently known subgroup variants. In the United States, laboratories should investigate with the manufacturers whether the kit is capable of detecting subtype O variants.

In the test, aliquots of sera are added to the wells of microtiter plates (solid phase) that have been coated with the synthetic viral peptides (antigens). If HIV antibody is present in the serum, it will bind to the antigen on the solid phase, forming an antigen–antibody complex. Following a wash step to remove unbound materials, an enzyme-conjugated anti-human IgG is dispensed into the wells. The conjugate binds to any antigen–antibody complex present and is retained by the solid phase following a second wash step. Bound conjugate is then detected by adding an enzyme substrate to the wells and measuring the rate of production of a colored product. If the rate of color production of the specimen is equal to or greater than a cut-off rate, the specimen is considered *reactive* for HIV antibody.

The screening test currently used is very sensitive for detecting HIV antibody in infected individuals. However, the test is not perfect and false-positive and false-negative results may occur.

At very early stages of infection, individuals may not yet have antibody levels high enough to produce a reaction and will therefore be falsely negative when tested for HIV infection by the ELISA. This period usually lasts 4 to 8 weeks after exposure but occasionally lasts as long as 26 weeks. Diagnosis of HIV infection in these individuals requires either a repeat test in a few weeks time or supplemental tests that detect either viral antigen (p24 antigen test) or nucleic acid (polymerase chain reaction, PCR).

The ELISA will also produce some false-positive results. Up to 25 percent of all repeat reactive ELISA results are from individuals who do not have HIV infection. Even after repeat testing, reactive results may occur in a small number of noninfected individuals. Most errors in testing are associated with mislabeling or sample contamination or carryover during some point in the process. Owing to the possibility of false-positive results, a reactive screen test cannot be considered conclusive evidence of HIV infection. A confirmatory test must be performed to verify true HIV status.

CONFIRMATORY TEST: WESTERN BLOT

The main purpose of confirmatory tests is to ensure that individuals who test positive on screening assays are not incorrectly regarded as HIV-infected. The Western blot is the most widely accepted confirmatory test for antibodies to HIV and is regarded by most authorities as the "gold standard" for verifying HIV results.

In the Western blot, individual viral proteins are separated into specific bands according to their molecular weights by electrophoresis through polyacrylamide gels. The bands are then transferred (blotted) onto nitrocellulose paper, which is cut into strips. The strips containing the separated viral antigens are now in a solid phase and the ELISA procedure is performed directly on the strip.

During incubation of test serum with the strip, specific antibodies to the viral components, if present, will bind to their respective antigens. If the serum sample contains antibodies to p24 and gp41, for example, they will bind only to specific antigens. Subsequent washing will remove unbound serum components. Conjugate addition, incubation, and washing then follow. The conjugate used is most often an anti-human IgG coupled to an enzyme, as in the ELISA screen. Finally, a precipitable substrate is added, and a colored precipitate forms on the nitrocellulose strip at the particular sites where specific antibodies have bound. Depending on the particular antibodies in the sample, band profiles will be produced.

The type of profile, that is, the combination and intensity of bands present, determines whether the individual is considered positive for antibodies to HIV. It is now universally accepted that a negative result means the absence of all bands on the blot, and that blots showing multiple bands corresponding to both virus core and envelope proteins should be considered positive for HIV antibodies. All other patterns of bands are considered indeterminate. An individual with an indeterminate result cannot be considered positive or negative until additional tests (p24 antigen, PCR, and/or recombinant ELISA) are performed, or until retesting is done at a future date.

The combined screening and confirmatory tests have excellent specificity (~99.9 percent) and sensitivity (~99.9 percent), but false-positive results may still occur. Most errors in testing are associated with mislabeling or carryover during some point in the process. The likelihood of a positive test being false is very low in groups with expected high seroprevalence and very high in individuals having no or little likelihood of HIV infection.

SUPPLEMENTAL TESTS

p24 Antigen

There are certain periods during HIV infection when viral core protein, p24 antigen, can be demonstrated in serum, thereby confirming infection. The p24 antigen test is useful in establishing HIV infection when early infection is suspected and the person is seronegative; in infants born to HIV-seropositive mothers; and in individuals who have tested negative or indeterminate for HIV antibodies but who are known to be at high risk and have symptoms of HIV infection. In HIV-positive individuals receiving antiviral therapy but not doing well, a positive p24 antigen test may indicate a lack of efficacy of the antiviral drug used and influence the decision to change the drug or its dosage.

The test to detect p24 antigen employs ELISA technology, but is somewhat modified because it is *antigen,* not antibody, that is being measured. In the assay, a specific monoclonal antibody to HIV p24 is attached to the solid phase. The test serum is added and if antigen is present in the serum, the antigen will attach to the monoclonal antibody in the solid phase. Following a wash step, conjugate is added and incubated. The conjugate in this case is an antibody to p24 antigen, coupled to an enzyme. A typical substrate reaction will usually detect the unknown antigen in the sample.

The p24 antigen test was not originally designed for testing serum and lacks sensitivity. While a positive p24 antigen result confirms HIV infection and may indicate an increased likelihood of progression to AIDS, a negative result does not preclude rapid progression.

HIV p24 Antigen with Immune Complex Dissociation

A major advance in HIV antigen detection has been the development of procedures used to break up immune complexes (essentially by destroying antibody) before testing for HIV antigen. These procedures are still under investigation, but show promise as relatively simple and accurate surrogate measurements of HIV viral load.

Saliva and Urine Testing for HIV Antibody

Testing saliva and/or urine for HIV antibody has many potential applications. The collection of saliva/urine is noninvasive, poses reduced biohazard risk to health care personnel, *and* has advantages in transportation. Both are currently being used as an epidemiologic tool in assessing the prevalence of HIV infection in specific populations, and offer advantages in testing populations in whom the collection of blood is not acceptable.

Currently in Canada, and more specifically in Ontario, testing saliva for HIV antibody may be performed for research purposes only. Kits used for HIV antibody testing must be authorized for sale in Canada by the Health Protection Branch, Health and Welfare Canada. To date no HIV kits have been authorized for testing saliva or urine. Patients may report being tested for HIV using saliva or urine by insurance companies. Such testing should *not* be considered diagnostic and if the patient requires HIV testing it should be repeated with a blood specimen.

The United States has recently authorized one product for HIV screening using saliva.

POLYMERASE CHAIN REACTION

The polymerase chain reaction (PCR) is an in vitro gene amplification technique that permits the selective amplification of HIV DNA segments directly in clinical specimens.

PCR begins with the denaturation of the target DNA, followed by the annealing of two primers that correspond to complementary strands of the target DNA and flank the region to be amplified. The hybrid formed between the primers and the target DNA creates a template–primer system recognized by a DNA polymerase. During the elongation step, the DNA polymerase replicates both strands of the DNA target sequence. Because the newly synthesized DNA by itself forms a template, repeated cycles of denaturation, annealing, and elongation result in an exponential increase in target sequence copies. After 30 rounds of PCR, a given target DNA sequence can be amplified over a million-fold, facilitating its detection with labeled probes.

Although not adapted for routine diagnosis of HIV infection, the technique has several uses, including detection of HIV gene sequences during early infection, before seroconversion; identifying the infection status of individuals with indeterminate serology results; and detecting infection in babies born to seropositive mothers.

While it is highly sensitive and specific, the PCR technique gives false-positive and negative results if not performed with the utmost of care. It is not a simple procedure, but requires careful and exact laboratory performance.

HIV RNA Polymerase Chain Reaction for Measurement of Viral Load

New tests are under development to quantify replicating virus. To date, these include an RNA PCR assay and a branch chain assay. The RNA PCR assay makes use of the enzyme reverse transcriptase to generate DNA from RNA present in the specimen. The resultant DNA is then amplified along with specific amounts of "designer DNA" as control. The amount of amplified DNA (using the designer DNA as internal control) is proportional to the amount of RNA in the original specimen. The Chiron branch chain DNA (bDNA) assay measures RNA directly by capturing it with DNA probes coated onto a micro-titer plate. Additional probes that are attached to "branched" DNA molecules sandwich the RNA. Each of the branches is a receptor for chemilumines-cent substrate, and the intensity of the reaction is propor-tional to the amount of RNA in the specimen. Both are in early stages of clinical trials and seem to be able to measure RNA across a range of 500 to 100,000 molecules per milliliter. To date, the assay has been shown to be a sensitive marker of the effectiveness of antiretroviral therapy in population studies. However, it is not yet clear whether the assay will be useful in assessing individual viral load, determining the effect of antiretroviral therapy, or predicting patient outcome and therefore have a role to play in patient management and care, although it is currently being used by some practitioners to monitor individuals.

These tests are not yet approved by the U.S. Food and Drug Administration. In Canada, the Roche Amplicor HIV-IPCR kit has recently been authorized by Health Canada on a clinical trial basis for specific circumstances. Criteria for PCR testing include detection of HIV genome in infants born to HIV-infected mothers, in persons with indeterminate HIV serology, and in other cases as discussed with laboratory staff. Consultation with laboratory staff is required before specimens are submitted. The PCR test is very expensive and must be carried out in conjunction with HIV culture and serology; all data during the clinical trial phase must be reported to Health Canada.

■ MEDICAL EVALUATION AND MANAGEMENT

Brian Cornelson, M.D., C.C.F.P.

Mary Fanning, M.D., Ph.D. F.R.C.P.C., F.A.C.P.

Ken Uffen, M.D., C.C.F.P.

The initial response of individuals to learning of a positive HIV result varies considerably. Some people may not be surprised with a positive result, knowing that they have engaged in activities that put them at risk for HIV. Some already have symptoms that have made them, or their physician, suspect HIV infection. Others may be completely taken aback and shocked with the result. Regardless of whether or not someone is expecting a positive result, it remains a traumatic experience to first learn of being HIV positive.

A person's initial response to learning of a positive HIV test result may be very emotional, especially if the news was unexpected. Others may be calm and matter-of-fact at first, until the initial shock wears off. However, adjustment to this new reality and its implications is a gradual process that may take weeks, months, or even years. The physician's role in the initial management of HIV-positive persons is not only to provide comprehensive medical follow-up, but also to provide or ensure social and emotional support, which may involve referrals to appropriate groups and agencies for specific concerns.

It it therefore vital that the physician recognize the complex and comprehensive challenge of dealing with HIV infection, which requires an organized, systematic, humane approach. It is impossible to do everything that is required in the first one or two visits, and indeed patients cannot remember and integrate all the advice, information, and instruction they require all at once. Physicians should schedule a series of half-hour appointments with patients over the first few weeks following serodiagnosis in order to work through the necessary investigations, education, and development of an ongoing management strategy.

Both physician and patient will be more comfortable knowing that they have an organized plan for implementing and monitoring all aspects of management. Using a set of flow sheets to manage information is helpful.

The following sections outline the essential elements in the initial management of the HIV-positive individual. Management is presented according to standard medical practice (i.e., history, physical examination, initial management, immunizations, initial investigations, and CD4 cell counts). If the family physician has conducted the pre- and post-test counseling, much of the history will already have been obtained. In most circumstances, the first item on the agenda will be a discussion of the person's reaction to the news of being HIV-positive—initial thoughts and emotions, and whether they were shared with anyone else—and answering questions that surface. Once general issues have been addressed, it is best to proceed with a more detailed history, physical examination, and management strategy according to the following guidelines. An open, sensitive, caring, nonjudgmental approach is essential.

INITIAL EVALUATION OF THE HIV-POSITIVE PATIENT

History

HIV History

The history should include the following questions:

- When was the person tested for HIV? Why was the test done? Were there any previous tests? When? What were the results?
- What risk activities has the person engaged in?
- What are the person's current risk activities? Provide education about prevention of transmission to *and* from their contacts.
- Try to estimate the approximate duration of HIV infection:
  —history of acute viremia symptoms (30 to 40 percent)?
  —when did they commence appropriate risk reduction (infection likely occurred before that date)?
- Contacts (sexual, injection drugs, children of infected women):
  —issues of informing and protecting contacts need to be addressed.
- Social factors:
  —living situation (alone, partner, family).
  —who knows about the diagnosis? Whom does the person plan to tell?
  —social supports (partner, family, friends).
  —employment status.
  —financial status.
  —who can help if patient becomes ill?

Past Medical History

In addition to the standard past medical history, specific information should include questions about the following:

- Tuberculosis: skin test status, exposure, socioeconomic status, illness, treatment, and duration of treatment.
- Syphilis: when diagnosed, treatment given, follow-up, and where records may be obtained.

- Herpes.
- Hepatitis B, C.
- Warts: anal/genital (occurrence, treatment, recurrences).
- Shingles.
- Pap smear, recurrent vaginal candidiasis.
- Immunization status: pneumococcus, tetanus and diphtheria, influenza, hepatitis A, B, hemophilus influenzae B.

Medication History

The medication history should include the following:

- Current and previous medications for HIV infection or its complications.
- Reasons for discontinuing medications (e.g., Zidovudine [AZT]).
- Other medications.
- Side effects and allergic reactions to medications.

Physical Examination

A complete physical examination should be done, focusing on areas particularly relevant to HIV infection, but also remembering to assess the patient generally, looking for other indicators of health, disease, or disability. Physical findings particularly relevant in HIV infection include the following:

- General: weight; temperature, pulse, respiratory rate if indicated.
- Retinal examination: cotton-wool spots, yellow-white retinal infiltrates (cytomegalovirus [CMV], toxoplasmosis), retinal hemorrhages (CMV) if CD4 count is <100.
- Oral examination: white plaques (candidiasis), white filaments on tongue (oral hairy leukoplakia), ulcers (herpes simplex virus [HSV], didanosine [ddI] use), purplish papules (Kaposi's sarcoma).
- Lymph nodes: generalized lymphadenopathy (HIV), rapid enlargement, or localized lymphadenopathy (tuberculosis, Mycobacterium avium complex [MAC], lymphoma, other tumors).
- Chest.
- Abdominal examination: hepatomegaly, splenomegaly (MAC, tuberculosis, lymphoma, histoplasmosis), perirectal ulcers (HSV, CMV).

- Skin:
  —Kaposi's sarcoma.
  —seborrheic dermatitis.
  —purpura (HIV-related idiopathic thrombocytopenic purpura [ITP]).
  —herpes-zoster, HSV.
  —drug eruption.
  —bacillary angiomatosis.
- Neurologic examination:
  —mental status: HIV-related cognitive impairment.
  —motor deficits: peripheral neuropathy, space-occupying
  CNS lesions, drug toxicities (ddI or zalcitabine [ddC]).

Initial Management

- Review patient's knowledge of implications of diagnosis.
- Review patient's supports: work, family, friends, etc.
- Outline general long-term effects of HIV infection.
- Outline measures to limit or manage complications of HIV
  infection.
- Emphasize importance of risk behavior reduction and/or
  elimination to lessen the risk of infecting others *and* to
  reduce the risk of being reinfected.
- Discuss importance of notifying known contacts.
- Outline short-term plans: investigations, etc.
- Offer sources of further information about HIV infection.
  Emphasize that the patient need only read what is of
  interest at the moment.
- Initiate immunizations (see Immunizations).
- Order initial investigations (see Initial Investigations).

Immunizations

- Tetanus and diphtheria (Td), if required (i.e., not within
  the past 10 years).
- Pneumococcus (Pneumovax-23®), if not previously given.
- Hepatitis B (Engerix-B®, Recombivax HB®), if HBsAg
  and anti-HBs negative, at 0, 1, and 6 months. Double
  dose increases effectiveness in immune-compromised
  individuals.
- *Haemophilus influenzae* B (ProHibIt, HibTitre).
- Influenza immunization every autumn as that year's serum
  becomes available.

Initial Investigations

- Complete blood cell count (CBC) (hemoglobin [Hb], hematocrit [Hct], white blood cell count [WBC] with differential, platelets, MCV).

- Liver function tests (alkaline phosphatase, [ALT] alanine transferase, [AST] aspartate transaminase, GGT, lactate dehydrogenase; protein/albumin); other routine (i.e., not related to HIV) screening (e.g., blood glucose, cholesterol, triglycerides, BUN, creatinine).

- HBsAg, anti-HBs if not known or not previously immunized.

- VDRL and confirmatory test (syphilis may be difficult to diagnose in someone who is HIV positive).

- Toxoplasmosis, CMV; cryptococcal antigen, Epstein-Barr virus *not* useful as routine screening tests.

- Pulmonary function tests and chest radiography as a baseline may be helpful; the changes of early *Pneumocystis carinii* pneumonia (PCP) can be subtle.

- Tuberculin skin test (Mantoux; 5TU PPD). If negative, repeat in 2 weeks and do anergy screen if CD4 count is <200. Consider induration of 2 mm as a positive reaction. If positive, no symptoms, and negative chest radiograph, start isoniazid (INH) 300 mg daily and continue for 9 months; monitor liver enzymes after first month. If the clinical or radiographic picture is suspicious for tuberculosis, isolate the patient and proceed with definitive investigations.

- CD4 cell counts (see below).

- The role of viral load measurement in routine care has not yet been established.

- In women, also perform Pap smear and swabs for culture and sensitivity and yeast. Manage abnormal Pap test results aggressively: if minor changes are noted, repeat in 3 months; if more significant changes or persistent minor changes are seen, refer for colposcopy. Treat yeast infections aggressively.

CD4 Cell Counts

CD4 cells (T-helper cells, T4 cells) are progressively depleted in HIV infection. CD4 cell counts are inexact, varying by as much as 25 percent at any one time and by laboratory and time of day when the blood is drawn. CD4 cell counts are also relatively poor indicators of immune function: some people have opportunistic infections when their CD4 counts are >200, others have never had any when their CD4 counts are ≤25. As well, they have no relation to other complications of HIV infection, such as malignancies or constitutional or neurologic symptoms. Nonetheless, they are useful as indicators of the need for further management, notably the use of antiretrovirals or opportunistic infection prophylaxis.

T-cell counts usually include the absolute number of CD4 cells, the CD4 percentage, the number of CD8 cells, and the CD4/CD8 ratio. CD8 cells (T-suppressor cells, T8 cells) are often elevated earlier in the infection. A drop in CD8 cells may precede a drop in CD4 cells.

A T-cell count should be done initially, and repeated in 3 months if the result is well within normal (e.g., >600). If it is less than this, it can be repeated at monthly intervals until two or three counts are obtained, to be reasonably sure of the range (because the counts are relatively variable).

As a rough guideline pending T-cell count result (which can take 1 to 2 weeks), if the absolute lymphocyte count is >1500, the CD4 count is probably >200. If the absolute lymphocyte count is <1500, the CD4 count is probably <500.

THE "TYRANNY OF THE T-CELLS". Unfortunately, many patients come to focus all their hopes and fears on the results of their CD4 cell counts. They are elated if the number is up, depressed if it is down. It is important to remind people that the numbers vary by 25 percent under the best of circumstances, that many other temporary factors can influence the numbers, and that it is the *trend,* rather than the absolute number, that is crucial. It is also essential that people know that CD4 cell counts are *not* an accurate reflection of the functioning of the immune system, and that there are many other aspects of HIV infection that have nothing to do with T-cells. In fact, T-cell counts should simply be used as indicators for initiating antiretroviral therapy or opportunistic infection prophylaxis. The physician can avoid colluding with this "tyranny" by de-emphasizing the results, by explaining their limitations, by *not* ordering them unless an important management change is anticipated as a result of testing, and by focusing on other, more significant but less-well measured, parameters such as energy level, weight, and the absence of specific symptoms.

ROUTINE MONITORING OF *ASYMPTOMATIC* HIV-POSITIVE PATIENTS

Once the initial management is completed, the next phase is the routine monitoring of patients with HIV infection. The asymptomatic individual with a CD4 cell count of ≥300 probably only needs to be seen every 3 to 6 months. When seeing an asymptomatic individual for follow-up, the routine described below will help to focus the visits.

History

- Energy/fatigue, weight/appetite, sleeping, mood, headache, visual changes, oral complaints, difficulty swallowing, cough, difficulty breathing, diarrhea, numbness, weakness, skin complaints, mood.

- Social functioning: support from spouse/partner, family, friends, agencies, etc.; work/school; financial concerns.

Physical Examination

- As emphasized in the initial assessment, paying particular attention to symptomatic areas or areas of previous difficulty.

- Annual complete health examination, focusing on *non*-HIV health assessment (people with HIV infection also get non-HIV health problems!).

LABORATORY INVESTIGATIONS

In the asymptomatic HIV-positive individual taking no medications, routine laboratory monitoring should include a CBC (to monitor the development of anemia) and a T-cell count every 3 to 6 months to track the need to start thinking about specific antiretroviral therapy or opportunistic infection prophylaxis.

Management

The timing of medication for HIV infection is the next major hurdle to be faced. It is best to start talking about this before actually recommending specific therapy. As CD4 cells start to fall to threshold levels (e.g., 200 for PCP prophylaxis), the need to prevent opportunistic infection must be discussed with the patient. When to initiate antiretrovirals and which one(s) to recommend continues to be a controversial and constantly evolving subject. Recent literature and local authorities should be consulted.

ROUTINE MONITORING OF *SYMPTOMATIC* HIV-POSITIVE PATIENTS

"Symptomatic" refers to HIV-infected individuals who have developed specific HIV-related problems and those who have been started on antiretroviral therapy or opportunistic infection prophylaxis. In addition to the standard monitoring outlined above for asymptomatic individuals, these patients should be monitored as follows:

History

- Inquire about any difficulties with or side-effects from the medications taken.

- Emphasize questions relating to specific complications (e.g., difficulty breathing, visual changes, diarrhea, nutrition, mental changes).

- Inquire about support from others, whether they still feel able to work, if their (biological) family is aware of their condition, if they have considered making a living will and organizing power of attorney.

Physical Examination

- Monitor weight closely, also oral cavity, skin, mood, mental status, and neurologic functioning.

Investigations

Patients on medication should be monitored according to the requirements of the particular medications:

- Zidovudine:
  —baseline Hb, WBC with differential, platelets, reticulocytes; BUN, creatinine; creatine kinase [CK]; AST, ALT, LDH, alkaline phosphatase, bilirubin; vitamin B_{12} and red blood cell folate.
  —after first 2 weeks and monthly thereafter: CBC, liver function tests.
  —every 3 months: CD4 count, CK.

- Didanosine (ddI), zalcitabine (ddC), stavudine (d4t), lamivudine (3TC):
  —baseline, after first 2 weeks and monthly: Hb, WBC with differential, platelets, reticulocytes; BUN, creatinine;

AST, ALT, LDH, alkaline phosphatase, bilirubin; uric acid, amylase, triglycerides.
—every 3 months: CD4 count.

- Saquinavir, Ritonavir, Indinavir:
  —baseline, after first 2 weeks and monthly: Hb, WBC with differential, platelets, reticulocytes; BUN, creatinine; AST, ALT, LDH, alkaline phosphatase, bilirubin, amylase.
  —every 3 months: CD4 count, CK.
  —Indinavir—monthly urinalysis
  Note: Resistance to AZT, ddI, and ddC has been observed and may contribute to clinical failure.

  3TC and Neveripine should not be used as monotherapy because of the rapid emergence of resistance.

  The use of viral load measurements for monitoring drug therapy has not been approved and no clear guidelines exist to advise those who wish to follow these tests.

Management

Annual immunizations must be administered. Non-HIV-related health problems can occur and should not be overlooked.

ANTIRETROVIRAL THERAPY

Zidovudine (AZT, Azidothymidine, Retrovir)

Zidovudine is a nucleoside analog that inhibits HIV reverse transcriptase. It is recommended for people with AIDS or those who are infected with HIV and have CD4 counts <200, as well as individuals with CD4 counts between 200 and 500 with symptoms of HIV infection. Treatment decisions should be individualized for asymptomatic individuals with CD4 counts between 200 and 500 because the data regarding its benefits in this group are contradictory. Treatment of individuals with CD4 counts >500 did not slow progression to AIDS or prolong survival. Treatment of acute retroviral syndrome may improve the clinical course. Treatment of HIV-infected pregnant women markedly reduces HIV transmission to their infants.

Zidovudine comes in 100-mg tablets and was originally prescribed as 2 tablets q4h around the clock, providing a total dose of 1200 mg/day but forcing people to wake up in the night every 4 hours. These dosages are toxic to bone marrow and almost everybody developed a rather significant megaloblastic anemia. The current dosing regimen is 100 mg 5 times/day. At these dosages almost everyone becomes megaloblastic but very few become significantly anemic. A variety of other dosage regimens, such as 200 mg q8h or reduced dosages of 100 mg QID or 100 mg TID, may be prescribed.

The anemia associated with zidovudine does not respond to supplemental folate or vitamin B_{12} administration, although it is more prevalent in patients who had low pretreatment levels.

Recombinant human erythropoietin is effective in a small number of people who become anemic and symptomatic from that anemia. It is recommended if the blood erythropoietin level is <500.

It is still not known whether the myopathy that is reportedly related to zidovudine is in fact just a natural consequence of HIV infection. This myopathy is an annoying muscular ache or pain with weakness, which may become debilitating and be associated with elevations of the CK enzyme. Discontinuing the zidovudine may not improve the symptoms.

Patients on zidovudine should be seen at least monthly and have general chemistry and hematologic evaluations monthly at first, then every 2 months, if stable.

Fingerpricks/Occupational Exposure

At the time of writing, the Centers for Disease Control in Atlanta had not yet changed its recommendation of offering to treat occupational exposures (i.e., fingerpricks in surgery) with zidovudine 1200 mg/day starting within 24 hours of exposure and continuing for 6 weeks. However, failures have been reported with this regimen. With the approval of a new class of drugs (proteases), new prophylactic recommendations are expected in 1996.

Didanosine (ddI, Dideoxyinosine, Videx)

Didanosine works by a mechanism similar to that of zidovudine. Indications are the following:

- Intolerance to zidovudine at 500 mg/day or lower, or
- Progression of clinical disease despite zidovudine treatment.
- CD4 count below 200.

Didanosine has also been used in combination with zidovudine. Dosages are as follows:

- for patients >75 kg: 2 × 150-mg tablets BID
- for patients 50 to 74 kg: 2 × 100 mg tablets BID
- for patients <50 kg: 1 × 100 mg and 1 × 25 mg tablet BID

Didanosine produces painful chronic peripheral neuropathies that give a mild stocking-and-glove pattern of discomfort to almost everyone and are enough to preclude its use in 20 to 30% of individuals. It is a buffered preparation and consequently decreases the absorption of ketoconazole, itraconazole, and dapsone, and must therefore be given 2 hours before these drugs. Because of the aluminum and calcium salts in the buffer, didanosine precludes the concomitant use of tetracyclines.

However, didanosine does not potentiate the myelosuppressive effects of ganciclovir (as does zidovudine), and consequently it is commonly used in conjunction with ganciclovir when patients develop CMV infections.

Zalcitabine (ddC, Dideoxycytidine, HIVID)

Zalcitabine is similar to ddI. It is approved as combination therapy with zidovudine when CD4 counts are <300. The usual dose is 0.75 mg TID, and because of drug interactions, zalcitabine should be stopped or at least more closely monitored when giving metronidazole, didanosine, or disulfiram (Antabuse). Patients should be monitored carefully for pancreatitis if IV pentamidine is administered. Other complications include peripheral neuropathy, rash, fever, stomatitis, and esophageal ulceration.

Staduvine (d4T, Zerit)

Staduvine is another HIV reverse transcriptase inhibitor that has some activity against zidovudine-resistant strains. It is approved for treatment of individuals intolerant of other nucleoside analogs, those who have disease progression (clinical or CD4 decline) while on other treatments, or those who have received prolonged prior zidovudine therapy.

The dosages are as follows:

- 40 mg BID for patients ≥60 kg.
- 30 mg BID for patients <60 kg.

Dosage should be modified in patients with reduced creatinine clearance.

The major toxicity is dose-related peripheral neuropathy, which occurs in 19-24% of patients with advanced disease and 14% of those with less advanced HIV disease.

Lamivudine (3TC, Epivir)

Lamivudine is an HIV reverse transcriptase inhibitor. Rapid resistance develops when it is used as monotherapy. It has recently been approved in combination with zidovudine for patients with advanced HIV disease and for previously untreated patients with CD4 counts ≤300. Patients in these categories sustained higher increases of CD4 cell counts on AZT-3TC combination than in comparison monotherapy groups. There is no information on the effect of this combination on clinical progression or survival. It is given at a dosage of 300 mg BID and is generally well tolerated, with major side effects of nausea, diarrhea, anemia, low white blood cell count, pancreatitis (especially in children on prior nucleoside therapy and neuropathy). Dose reduction is recommended in renal failure.

Neveripine

Neveripine is a non-nucleoside reverse transcriptase inhibitor (NNRTI) recently approved for use only in combination with a reverse transcriptase inhibitor and possibly a second agent, e.g., aprotease inhibitor. This drug and others in its class are characterized by rapid emergence of HIV resistance when used as monotherapy.

Saquinavir (Invirase)

Saquinavir is in a new class of drugs that inhibit HIV protease activity and are effective against viral strains resistant to nucleoside analogs. It is recommended in combination with other antiretrovirals for treatment of patients with advanced disease and no prior zidovudine use. Combination therapy with zidovudine is recommended in naive patients and with HIVID if previous treatment with zidovudine was administered. It is given at a dosage of 600 mg q8h. Adverse events such as diarrhea, nausea, and abdominal discomfort are generally mild.

Ritonavir (Norvir)

Ritonavir is an HIV protease inhibitor which has been approved in combination with nucleoside analogues or as monotherapy for the treatment of HIV when therapy is warranted. Treatment in advanced disease has demonstrated a reduction in mortality and disease progression over 6 months. In less advanced disease ritonavir led to sustained increases of CD4 count and decreases in viral load.

Ritonavir should be taken with meals at a dosage of 600 mg twice daily. Dose escalation may reduce symptoms of nausea; 300 mg twice daily for 1 day, 400 mg twice daily for 2 days, 500 mg twice daily for 1 day and then 600 mg twice daily thereafter. Side effects are gastrointestinal (nausea, diarrhea, vomiting, anorexia, abdominal pain and taste perversion) which, with the exception of diarrhea, are amplified by combination with zidovudine and neurologic (circumoral and peripheral paresthesias). Numerous serious drug interactions occur and the drug label should be reviewed or a pharmacist consulted when prescribing other medications.

Indinavir (Crixivan)

Indinavir is an HIV protease inhibitor approved on the basis of surrogate endpoints for treatment of HIV infection when antiretroviral therapy is warranted. Indinavir alone or in combination led to sustained decreased viral RNA load and increased CD4 counts compared to zidovudine mono-therapy. These changes were more marked in previously zidovudine naive patients with mean CD4 counts of 145 and 254, than in patients previously on zidovudine (median time—30.9 months). The recommended dosage is 800 mg (two 400 mg capsules) orally every 8 hours on an empty stomach. Adverse events of note are nephrolithiasis which occurs infrequently and should lead to temporary interruption of treatment (1-3 days). Adequate hydration is recommended for all patients receiving indinavir. Bilirubin elevation occurs more frequently sometimes with elevations of serum transaminases. The dosage should be lowered in patients with hepatic insufficiency. Serious drug interactions occur with terfenadine, astemizole, cisapride, triazolam, and midazolam and these drugs should not be co-administered. Rifabutin dosage should be lowered and Rifampin avoided entirely. Ketocorazole leads to increased levels of indinavir. Indinavir dosage should be reduced if the patient is on ketoconazole.

Acyclovir

Use of acyclovir remains controversial, but unpublished data from the 1992 Amsterdam conference suggest that early studies presented in Stockholm in 1988 were correct in that high doses (800 mg 5 times/day) may augment the anti-HIV action of antiretrovirals. In those receiving acyclovir mortality decreased after 1 year but CMV infection did not decrease.

Therapy Summary

1. CD4 count 200 to 500, asymptomatic: zidovudine alone or in combination with didanosine, zalcitabine, lamivudine, or proteases, or no therapy.

   CD4 200 to 500, symptomatic: zidovudine 200 mg

TID or 100 mg 5 times/day, or in combination with didanosine, zalcitabine, lamivudine, saquinavir, ritonavir or indinavir.

2. CD4 <200: zidovudine alone or in combination with didanosine, zalcitabine, lamivudine, saquinavir, ritonavir or indinavir.

   With a significant drop in the CD4 count or progression of disease, change zidovudine to or add didanosine, lamuvidine, saquinavir, ritonavir or indinavir (see previous sections for dosage).

3. Zidovudine intolerance: switch to didanosine, or staduvine.

4. Didanosine intolerance: consider zalcitabine or staduvine (similar toxicity).

5. Consider acyclovir 800 mg 5 times/day.

   Note: These recommendations are expected to change as new information about combination therapies becomes available over the next one to two years.

OPPORTUNISTIC INFECTION PROPHYLAXIS

With CD4 counts ≤200, ≤20 percent or prior PCP, prophylaxis against recurrent PCP includes the following:

- Trimethoprim-sulfamethoxazole (TMP-SMX) 1 DS tablet once* or twice daily given 2, 3, or 7 days/week.

- If toxicity is evident with TMP-SMX, aerosolized pentamidine (Respigard II) 300 mg/month.

- Dapsone 50 to 100 mg daily, or 100 mg 2 times/week.

- Pyrimethamine 50 mg plus dapsone 100 to 200 mg 2 times/week.

Other drugs, such as IV pentamidine 300 mg/month, Atovaquone, or Fansidar, can be used as alternatives if the above regimens cannot be tolerated.

With CD4 counts ≤100 prophylaxis of toxoplasmosis or cryptococcal infection may have little or no clinical impact.

- For toxoplasmosis: consider pyramethamine 25 to 50/day or pyrimethamine 25 to 50 mg/day and sulfadiazine 500 to 1000 mg/day.

---

*Preferred regimen. 1 DS tablet daily, 7x/week

- For cryptococcal infection consider fluconazole 100 mg daily.

- For MAC: clarithromycin 250 mg twice/day, rifabutin 300 mg/day, or azithromycin 500 mg 3 times/week.

- Tuberculosis: isoniazid 300 mg daily.

Suggested Readings

Drugs for AIDS and associated infections. Med Lett 1995; 37:87–94.

Gallant JE, Moore RD, Chaisson RE. Prophylaxis for opportunistic infections in patients with HIV infection. Ann Intern Med 1994; 120:932–44.

Sande MA, Carpenter CCJ, Cobbs CG, et al. Antiretroviral therapy for adult HIV-infected patients. Recommendations from a state-of-the-art conference. JAMA 1993; 270:2583–89.

USPHS/IDSA guidelines for the prevention of opportunistic infections in persons infected with human immunodeficiency virus: A summary. MMWR 1995; 44 (RR-8):1–34.

▆▆▆ OCCUPATIONAL EXPOSURE

Susan Shurtleff, R.N., C.I.C.

PRACTICES TO PROTECT HEALTH CARE WORKERS FROM OCCUPATIONAL EXPOSURE TO BLOOD AND BODILY FLUIDS

Hospitals should employ an approved system of precautions for infection control purposes. There should be an Infection Control Manual on each hospital unit and in each department outlining the system.

The principles of INFECTION CONTROL PRECAUTIONS include the following:

1. Effective appropriate hand washing at *all* times.

   - Wash hands *before:*
     —all sterile and/or invasive procedures.
     —eating.

   - Wash hands *after:*
     —direct patient care.
     —handling waste.
     —handling soiled linen.
     —handling soiled equipment.
     —contact with any body substance.
     —glove removal.

2. Appropriate handling and disposal of sharps and sharp objects.

  - Never bend or break needles.
  - Discard *all* used sharps at point of use in designated container.
  - Discard your own used sharps.
  - Do not recap; if you must recap, use a *safe* recapping method.

3. Use protective barrier equipment (mask, gown, goggle, or face shield) to prevent exposure of skin and mucous membranes to bodily substances and certain infectious diseases.

4. Consider all patient specimens infectious and handle accordingly.

5. Contain and handle accordingly all soiled reusable articles, waste, and linen.

6. Resuscitation devices are to be used for *all* situations requiring resuscitation. Resuscitation devices should be available in each patient's room and in other designated areas throughout the hospital.

PROCEDURE FOR MANAGEMENT OF A SHARP INJURY, OR MUCOUS MEMBRANE OR NONINTACT SKIN EXPOSURE

Note: All employees, including medical staff, should report all sharps injuries and exposures to the Department of Occupational Health or other designated department if Occupational Health is closed.

Procedure for Management

1. Flush exposed/injured area with fresh running water for 5 minutes.

2. Report to Occupational Health or other designated department.

3. Employees sustaining injuries/exposures from a known HIV-positive source may wish to consider zidovudine (AZT)* prophylaxis. Zidovudine prophylaxis should be started as soon as possible after the exposure.

Note: The efficacy of zidovudine has not been proven. More information regarding prophylaxis will be available in 1996.

4. Employees sustaining injuries/exposures from a source in whom the HIV status is not known should approach the attending physician or the designated individual to obtain consent for testing. An HIV test may only be ordered on a patient after informed consent has been obtained and pre-/post-test counseling has been completed/arranged.

Suggested Reading

Sande MA, Carpenter CCJ, Cobbs CG, et al. Antiretroviral therapy for adult HIV-infected patients. Recommendations from a state-of-the-art conference. JAMA 1993; 270:2583–89.

Gerberding J. Management of occupational exposures to blood-borne viruses. NEJM 1995; 332:No. 7, 444–451.

Women and HIV

Sharon Walmsley, M.D., F.R.C.P.C.

EPIDEMIOLOGY

Worldwide, approximately one-third of cases of HIV infection have occurred in women. An increasing proportion of new cases in North America is occurring in women. In Canada, the major risk factor for women is heterosexual sex, although intravenous drug use is another important risk factor which is the most common in the United States.

MEDICAL ISSUES

As women frequently do not perceive themselves to be at risk, they often do not present until a child or infected partner has been diagnosed with AIDS. Early signs and symptoms of HIV in women can include recurrent oral or vulvovaginal candidiasis, herpes-zoster, diarrhea, weight loss, and fatigue.

Pneumocystis carinii pneumonia (PCP) remains the commonest presenting AIDS-defining illness in women. Wasting syndrome and esophageal candidiasis are other common presenting symptoms. Kaposi's sarcoma is seen infrequently in women with HIV, and when it does occur, it typically occurs late and is very aggressive.

When controlling for CD4 count, access to medical care, and treatment, the survival for women living with HIV is similar to that for men.

The medical management of HIV (prevention and treatment of opportunistic infections and antiviral treatment) in women is similar to that in men, although good pharmacokinetic and toxicity studies to confirm that drugs should be used in the same doses are lacking. Rifampin can interfere with the metabolism of oral contraceptives and decrease their effectiveness.

GYNECOLOGIC ISSUES

Women living with HIV must be monitored for other sexually transmitted diseases, including gonorrhea, chlamydia, herpes simplex, and trichomonas. These gynecologic infections may be clinically silent. The prevalence of cervical and vaginal infections with the human papilloma virus (HPV) is increased in women with HIV, especially as the CD4 count declines. It has been estimated that approximately 25 percent of asymptomatic HIV-infected women have such infection; this figure rises to approximately 50 percent in those with more advanced disease. HPV is considered a major risk factor for cervical abnormalities. Cervical dysplasia and invasive cervical cancer are increased in women living with HIV. Invasive cervical cancer is now considered to be an AIDS-defining illness for women. Because of the increased risk of dysplasia and cancer, Pap smears are recommended at least every 6 months, and if abnormalities are found, the patient should be referred to a gynecologist for colposcopy and/or biopsy. The optimal management of dysplasia and carcinoma in women with HIV is uncertain, but early studies have suggested that they may not respond adequately to standard therapy with cryotherapy or ablative techniques. Recurrent candidal vulvovaginitis is a frequent complication in women with HIV and may be managed with topical antifungal creams (clotrimazole, nystatin) or oral azole drugs as they are in non-HIV infected women. Long-term suppressive therapy with azoles may be required in those cases with frequent recurrences. Menstrual abnormalities, including missed menses, intermenstrual spotting, and early menopause, are frequently reported. The contributions of HIV, malnutrition, drugs, and intercurrent illness are unclear.

OBSTETRICS

HIV infection does not adversely affect fertility. Pregnancy in itself does not appear to alter the natural course of HIV infection. Many women living with HIV chose to become pregnant. The risk of maternal fetal transmission of HIV is approximately 25 percent. This risk is increased with more advanced maternal illness, likely a reflection of increased viral loads.

Protocol ACTG 076, recently published in the *New England Journal of Medicine,* has demonstrated in a placebo-controlled trial that zidovudine (AZT) use in pregnancy can decrease the risk of maternal fetal transmission from 25 percent to 8 percent. In this study, women who were pregnant and had CD4 counts >200 between 14 and 34 weeks of gestation were given zidovudine at a dose of 100 mg q4h during their pregnancy, as an intravenous drip during labor and delivery (2 mg/kg load over 1 hour followed by 1 mg/kg/hour drip for the duration of labor and delivery), and the neonates were given zidovudine syrup at a dose of 2 mg/kg q6h for the first 6 weeks of life.

Although cohort studies have suggested possible decreased risk of transmission following cesarean section, this procedure cannot be routinely recommended. Other invasive procedures, such as episiotomy, use of scalp electrodes, scalp pH, and invasive monitoring, should be avoided where possible.

Breast feeding poses an incremental risk of transmission of approximately 15 percent. In North America, where safe forms of milk supplementation are available, breast feeding is not recommended for HIV-infected women and their children.

Pregnant women with CD4 counts >200 or 20 percent are at risk for pneumocystis carinii pneumonia (PCP) during pregnancy and should be given prophylaxis. Trimethoprim-sulfamethoxazole is the recommended agent.

PSYCHOSOCIAL ISSUES

Women living with HIV do not have a natural support group and often feel isolated in their disease. Physicians caring for women have to be aware of feelings of shame, guilt, despair, and isolation. Women are frequently the primary care givers for an infected child or partner, thereby having many responsibilities, and often put their own health or medical care last. Some women who test positive are at risk of physical or verbal violence from their partners upon diagnosis. Care givers must be aware of this possibility during pre- and post-test counseling and follow-up of these women. Many women do not have the power to negotiate safe-sex practices with their partners.

Suggested Readings

Chin J. Epidemiology: Current and future dimensions of the HIV/AIDS pandemic in women and children. Lancet 1990; 336:221–4.

Connor EM, Sperling RS, Gelber R, et al. Reduction of maternal-infant transmission of Human Immunodeficiency Virus type I with zidovudine treatment. N Engl J Med 1994; 331:1173–80.

Dunn DT, Newell ML, Mayaux MJ, et al. Mode of delivery and vertical transmission of HIV-1: A review of prospective studies. J AIDS 1994; 7:106–6.

Hankins CA, Handley MA. HIV disease and AIDS in women: Current knowledge and a research agenda. J AIDS 1992; 5:957–71.

Hankins CA, Lamont JA, Handley MA. Cervicovaginal screening in women with HIV infection: A need for increased vigilance? Can Med Assoc J 1994; 150:681–6.

Maiman M, Fruchter RG, Serur E, et al. Recurrent cervical intraepithelial neoplasia in Human Immunodeficiency Virus-seropositive women. Obstet Gynecol 1993; 82:170–4.

Phillips AN, Antunes F, Stergious G, et al. A sex comparison of rates of new AIDS-defining disease and death in 2554 AIDS cases. AIDS 1994; 8:831–5.

Heroin, Crack Cocaine, and HIV Infection

AN APPROACH TO ADDICTED HIV PATIENTS

Philip Berger, M.D., C.C.F.P., F.C.F.P.
Richard Fralick, M.D., F.R.C.P.

Addiction to mood-altering chemicals or chemical dependence can be characterized as loss of control over use, craving and compulsion, continued use despite adverse consequences, and denial that the dependence exists despite definitive evidence to the contrary.

THE DUAL PROBLEM OF HIV AND ADDICTION

The combination of HIV infection and addiction gives rise to special problems that complicate the provision of health care to persons afflicted with both conditions:

- Numerous physical and psychological conditions that arise directly from drug addiction.[1]
- A higher incidence (than with addiction or HIV alone) of sexually transmitted diseases, all types of viral hepatitis, bacterial pneumonia and endocarditis, tuberculosis, other retroviral infections, and certain cancers.[1]
- The increased risk of transmission of HIV and other sexually transmitted diseases to the public from HIV-infected addicts.[2]
- Management of HIV-related conditions that cause pain.
- Limited or nonexistent family and social support.

- Severe shortage of substance abuse rehabilitation and treatment programs.

The evidence concerning the effect of continuing substance abuse on the course of HIV infection is contradictory; no definite statement can be made about whether substance abuse itself accelerates HIV infection. However, HIV infection can act as a stressor or trigger for continued substance abuse.

RANGE OF PROBLEMS

The prevalence (mostly injection use) of heroin use in metropolitan Toronto is conservatively estimated at 14,000 people.[3] Thirty-four percent of AIDS cases in the United States have been attributed to injection use (through users or their sexual contacts).[1] Heroin can be smoked or snorted but is usually administered through intravenous injection.

The prevalence of lifetime cocaine use in Ontario is estimated to be 435,000 people.[9] The prevalence of lifetime crack cocaine use is 53,000 people, representing a marked explosion of use in the past year.

Cocaine can be snorted, smoked or injected intravenously. Crack cocaine is the smokable form of cocaine base also known as *rock*. It is a low-cost drug that was popularized in the mid-1980s, especially among young adults and street youth from lower socioeconomic groups. The inhalation of crack cocaine leads to rapid access into the blood stream with intense euphoria followed by prolonged withdrawal symptoms and craving for *more* drug. In U.S. centers like New York and Miami, particularly poor inner city communities, there is a high risk for HIV infection among young smokers of crack cocaine between the ages of 18 and 29 years, and especially among women who have sex in exchange for money or drugs. Crack cocaine is promoting the heterosexual transmission of HIV.[2]

HISTORY AND PHYSICAL EXAMINATION

Identification of HIV-infected persons who use drugs is paramount. A thorough, empathetic and noncritical history should be taken and should include the type of drugs used, the method and pattern of use, and previous treatment programs. Physicians should be familiar with the drug user's vocabulary.[4] Use of street terms in history taking can set an addict at ease. An inquiry into current and past medical and psychological problems (including legal and prison history) will assist in developing a comprehensive treatment program.

Physical examination should be directed toward current and past evidence of cellulitis, abscess, and points of injection of needles. Signs of current intoxication with drugs should be documented, including obvious sedation, changes in pupils, sweating, rapid heat rate, elevated blood pressure, or agitation. Withdrawal signs, including mood changes, excessive tearing, and rapid heart rate, should be recorded.

Urine drug screening can form part of the assessment of the HIV-infected addict providing that the patient provides fully informed consent for such testing.[5]

TREATMENT

General

Treatment begins with a compassionate, nonjudgmental approach. There are a variety of treatment options. Harm reduction is one important treatment approach. It can reduce or control the drug intake, to the extent possible. It will minimize or eliminate the risks associated with drug use. Abstinence is not, however, the goal. The success of harm reduction is measured in reduced drug use. A notable example is the use of methadone for heroin addiction.

In the hospital and in the community, there are times when the prescribing of narcotics and/or benzodiazepines are necessary (e.g., treating chronic pain or insomnia). However, some patients require strict limits on the amounts prescribed (Fig. 5–1).

Another treatment strategy is the use of needle exchange programs. These are designed to reduce the risk of infection, notably to HIV as well as hepatitis B, among drug users. However, these programs also provide education on the risks associated with drug use and emphasize the importance of safer sex practices. Condoms are provided along with clean needles. Often such programs invite people/users into the health care system, where further treatment options then become available.

Heroin

The use of methadone as part of a comprehensive heroin addiction treatment program is highly successful and unsurpassed in effectiveness by any other treatment approach. Methadone is an orally administered addictive

This contract of agreement re: the prescribing of pain killers and benzodiazepines is for (name). His/her doctor is Dr. _____ .

1. Dr. _____ will prescribe (specify drugs) at specific doses. He is the sole prescriber. The doses will be decided on through discussion with Dr. _____ . I will adhere to the doses. If the amount prescribed is not enough it is my responsibility to call Dr. _____ .

2. If Dr. _____ is away, another doctor will be designated to prescribe medications.

3. Prescriptions will be written one week at a time. The pharmacist will be instructed to dispense the meds on Monday, Wednesday, and Friday.

4. (name) _____ , you are responsible to safeguard your meds at all times. Lost or stolen meds will not be replaced.

5. Random drug screens may be required at any time. A positive urine for an unauthorized substance will be grounds for discharge from Dr. _____'s care. If you see another doctor without my agreement that is also grounds for discharge from my care.

Signed:

_____   _____
(Patient)   (Witness)

_____
Date

Copy: Pharmacist

raf/

■■■■ FIGURE 5-1
Patient Contract Detailing Patient's and Doctor's Responsibilities with Regard to Prescription Pain Killer and Benzodiazepine Use

narcotic first synthesized in Germany during the Second
World War. Methadone eliminates heroin withdrawal symptoms, prevents cravings once addicts are abstinent, and
blocks the effects of heroin if addicts relapse. Many studies
indicate that methadone programs dramatically reduce the
transmission of HIV in addicted populations and reduce
crime with its associated police, judicial, legal aid, and
prison costs.[6] Methadone programs promote employment
and family stability. By any measure methadone programs
report up to an 85 percent success rate in treatment of heroin
addiction compared to 25 percent in abstinence programs.

Ontario physicians who wish to prescribe methadone must
first receive approval from the College of Physicians &
Surgeons of Ontario and acquire a license for each patient
using methadone from the Bureau of Drug Surveillance,
Health Canada. Guidelines for the prescribing of methadone
are available from the Bureau of Drug Surveillance and
physicians must fully comply in order to maintain a
prescribing license for each patient.[7,8]

In the United States, methadone is provided through special licensed and regulated methadone clinics and physicians registered with the Drug Enforcement Agency (DEA).

Crack Cocaine

Although the tricyclic antidepressant desipramine decreased the amount of cocaine use in outpatients who had
been studied, there is no definite drug with methadone-like
properties for the treatment of cocaine addiction.[10] There are
several drugs available for the pharmacologic treatment of
cocaine, but these are best considered experimental.[1]

It is often essential to remove crack cocaine users from
their home environment. Attention must be given to safety
(away from other drug users) as well as shelter and adequate
food. Detoxification units can fill these needs and break the
cycle of continued, compulsive use. In initiating treatment it
is important to maintain the nonjudgmental approach with
emphasis on the benefits of drug abstinence and the adverse
health and social consequences of drug use. This type of
approach may increase patients' willingness to change their
current pattern of drug use.

It is important to identify long-term treatment opportunities. Options for cocaine treatment include individualized
counseling, attention to relapse prevention, and 12-step
programs like Cocaine Anonymous or Narcotics Anonymous. Written contracts between the physician and patient

often become necessary as a means of defining the limits and consequences of the patient's behavior.

Compliance

Continuing drug use will reduce compliance with HIV therapy. Former addicts may relapse as their HIV infection progresses and symptoms arise. However, compliance with HIV treatment regimens is good if treatment for substance abuse is part of a comprehensive plan for the HIV-infected addict. Therefore, addicts should be offered standard HIV therapies along with substance abuse treatment.

References

1. O'Connor PG, Selwyn PA, Schottenfield RS. Medical care for injection-drug users with human immunodeficiency virus infection. N Engl J Med 1994; 331:450–9.
2. Edin BR, Irwin KL, Faruque S, et al. Intersecting epidemics— crack cocaine use and HIV infection among inner-city young adults. N Engl J Med 1994; 331:1422–7.
3. Southtown Consulting, Inc. Heroin activity in Metropolitan Toronto: a study conducted for the Metropolitan Toronto Addictions Treatment Services Committee, July 7, 1995.
4. Drugs and Crime Data Center and Clearinghouse. Street Terms: Drugs and the Drug Trade. U.S. Department of Justice, Office of Justice Programs, Bureau of Justice Statistics, June 1994.
5. Kapur BM. Drug-testing methods and clinical interpretations of test results. Offprint. Bull Narcotics 1993; 45, No. 2.
6. Sorensen JL, Batki SL, Good P, Wilkinson K. Methadone maintenance program for AIDS-affected opiate addicts. J Substance Abuse Treatment 1989; 6:87–94.
7. Bureau of Drug Surveillance. The use of opioids in the management of opioid dependence. Minister of National Health and Welfare, Health & Welfare Canada, 1992.
8. Bureau of Drug Surveillance. Dispensing methadone for the treatment of opioid dependence. Minister of National Health and Welfare, Health & Welfare Canada, 1994.
9. Adlaf EM, Ivis FJ, Smart RG. Alcohol and other drug use among Ontario adults in 1994 and changes since 1977. Addiction Research Foundation, 1994.
10. Cotton P. "Harm reductions" approach may be middle ground. JAMA 1994; 271(21); 1641–5.

■ MEDICAL COMPLICATIONS OF HIV IN IV DRUG USERS

Mary Fanning, M.D., Ph.D., F.R.C.P.C., F.A.C.P.

In general, HIV progression in IV drug users is similar to that in patients with infection due to other modes of transmission. However, the special problems of nutritional deficiency, greater tendency to develop bacterial infection, and less access to and compliance with therapies that slow HIV disease may lead to accelerated progression.[1]

The clinical spectrum of HIV complications is very different in this group of patients and seems to represent an increase in the existing risk of IV drug-associated illnesses and associated mortality. Pyogenic bacterial infection, specifically bacterial endocarditis and pneumonia, are thus far more common in this group of patients and the risk increases with declining CD4 count. Tuberculosis, sexually transmitted diseases such as syphilis and human papillomavirus infection, hepatitis A, B, C, and D, human T-cell lymphotrophic virus type II infection, and rapidly progressive renal failure are also associated with HIV in this population.

Constitutional symptoms occur and may be due to either HIV infection or injection itself. The AIDS-defining illnesses that IV drug users present with are similar in their spectrum but differ greatly in their proportion from other individuals with HIV disease. In general, they experience more *Pneumocystis carinii* pneumonia, cryptococcal disease, wasting, and tuberculosis and less cytomegalovirus disease, Kaposi's sarcoma, and non-Hodgkin's lymphoma. The investigation of new symptoms in these patients should reflect the different disease spectrum they experience.

References

1. Alcabes P, Friedland G. Injection drug use and human immunodeficiency virus infection. Clin Infect Dis 1995; 20:1467–79.

6

Pediatric HIV

Susan M. King, M.D., C.M.

THE NEWBORN BORN TO AN HIV-INFECTED MOTHER

At birth, newborns of HIV-infected mothers are usually normal. There are no clinical features that distinguish infected from noninfected infants at birth. In recent prospective studies in the developed world, the transmission rate of HIV infection to infants of HIV-positive mothers has ranged from 14 to 33 percent.[1] However, in a study in which selected HIV-positive pregnant women were treated with zidovudine during pregnancy and intrapartum and then their infants treated postdelivery, the transmission rate was reduced to 8 percent.[2] For prophylaxis, the infant should receive from birth zidovudine syrup 2 mg/kg/dose QID for 6 weeks. If the mother is a hepatitis B virus carrier, HBsAg or HBeAg positive, then the infant should be given hepatitis B immunoglobulin and the hepatitis B vaccine series started. It is recommended that an HIV-positive mother not breast feed because of the potential for HIV transmission through breast milk.

Because all babies will be HIV antibody positive due to the passive transfer of antibodies from their mothers, the diagnosis of HIV infection is confirmed by testing for p24 antigen or HIV DNA sequences using polymerase chain reaction (PCR), or by HIV culture. These tests are usually performed by an HIV laboratory. Referral to a pediatric HIV program should be offered because the multidisciplinary teams in such programs have the resources to deal with the complexity of medical and psychosocial issues that face many of these families. All babies on zidovudine prophylaxis should have their hemoglobin checked at 1 month. Because *Pneumocystis carinii* pneumonia (PCP) occurs most frequently in infants 2 to 8 months of age and has a high mortality, PCP prophylaxis is recommended for all infants until their HIV status is determined.

HIV TESTS ON INFANTS

HIV antibody tests in infants are not diagnostic of HIV infection because of passive transfer of maternal antibodies. Maternal HIV antibodies have been detected in infants up to 18 months of age. Therefore, for all infants under 18 months of age, laboratory diagnosis is made by testing for viral antigen (p24) or HIV DNA sequences using PCR, or by HIV culture.

CONFIRMING THAT AN INFANT BORN TO AN HIV-POSITIVE MOTHER IS NOT INFECTED

The infant under 18 months of age can be determined to be uninfected if the infant has no HIV-associated symptoms, a normal CD4 count for age (Table 6–1) and two blood tests negative for HIV, with at least one of those tests taken after 6 months of age and each blood specimen tested by HIV PCR or HIV culture.

For the child older than 18 months of age, HIV antibody tests are interpreted as in adults.

Even if an infant is determined to be uninfected, that child should still be followed annually because of the psychosocial issues that may affect the health of a child born into a family with other members infected with HIV. Some issues in managing the affected child are disclosure of the diagnosis, chronic illness of a parent or sibling, and death of a parent or sibling.

MANAGEMENT OF THE HIV-INFECTED CHILD

In most situations the approach to management of HIV-infected children is similar to that of adults.[4] However, there are some important differences:

1. *History:* When taking the history it must be kept in mind that most children are not aware of their diagnosis, therefore approval of the parent or guardian should be obtained before discussing HIV/AIDS in front of the child. Management of children usually involves other family members, and many infected children are in families with more than one infected person, so information on the health and social situation of other family members is necessary.

TABLE 6-1

Interpretation of CD4 T-Lymphocyte Counts and Percentage of Total Lymphocytes

| Immunologic Category | AGE OF CHILD | | | | | |
| | <12 months | | 1–5 years | | 6–12 years | |
	µl	(%)	µl	(%)	µl	(%)
No evidence of suppression	≥1500	(≥25)	≥1000	(≥25)	≥500	(≥25)
Evidence of moderate suppression	750–1499	(15–24)	500–999	(15–24)	200–499	(15–24)
Severe suppression	<750	(<15)	<500	(<15)	<200	(<15)

From Centers for Disease Control and Prevention.[3]

2. *Physical Examination:* The general and specific findings to look for on physical examination of an adult with HIV infection also apply to children. In addition, in childhood, growth is an important measure of health, and measurement of height, weight, and head circumference is essential. The child's development (gross motor, fine motor, verbal and social skills) is a good measure of neurologic function.

3. *Investigations:* Laboratory evaluations are similar to those in adults, but the addition of varicella-zoster virus (VZV) titer to the initial investigations should be considered; if the child is susceptible to chicken pox then varicella-zoster immunoglobulin is recommended after an exposure to VZV. (If an HIV-infected child gets chicken pox, prompt treatment with acyclovir, IV or PO, is recommended.)

4. *Immunizations:* All HIV-infected children should receive routine childhood immunizations. For polio immunization, oral poliomyelitis vaccine should not be given to the child or family member; instead, inactivated poliomyelitis vaccine should be given. Annual influenza vaccination should be considered after 6 months of age and pneumococcal vaccine (Pneumovax) given once after the second birthday.

5. *Management:* Even if a child does not have full knowledge of the diagnosis, assent for treatment is still imperative. For many families, deciding how much to tell the child and when to tell the child that he or she is HIV-positive is very difficult for them. Until they have disclosed the diagnosis to the child, the family lives with secrecy and fear that their child will accidentally find out. The family should be encouraged to be truthful with their child, for example, by telling the child that there is a problem with his or her immune system, and then to add explanations as the child gets older and can understand more.

ANTIRETROVIRAL THERAPY IN CHILDREN

As in adults, antiretroviral therapy is recommended for patients with clinical or immunologic evidence of HIV-associated illness. The CD4 count is the most commonly used laboratory measure of immune function. The values are age dependent. Guidelines have been developed by the

Working Group on Antiretroviral Therapy: National Pediatric HIV Resource Center for using CD4 counts as indicators for starting antiretroviral therapy[5]:

Age	CD4 Cell Count
<1 year	<1750
1–2 years	<1000
2–6 years	<750
>6 years	<500

FEVER MANAGEMENT

The most common reasons for unscheduled visits of HIV-infected children are fever and cough. Young children with or without HIV infection have many febrile illness per year, most commonly caused by viral infection of the upper respiratory tract. There is no substitute for clinical judgment to decide which child has a serious illness and which one has benign one. The evaluation is similar to that in adults, with a decreasing threshold for investigation and empiric therapy as the patient's immune function deteriorates. The incidence of bacterial infections is higher in children than in adults with HIV. The bacterial pathogens and sites of infection are similar to those in immunocompetent children and therefore empiric antibiotic therapy is chosen accordingly.

If a febrile HIV-positive child, although immunocompromised, presents without an obvious source of infection and does not appear toxic, after a thorough assessment, the child may be observed without antibiotic therapy, provided the family situation allows for reliable follow-up in 24 hours.

PULMONARY SYMPTOMS

Lymphoid interstitial pneumonia (LIP) is the most common respiratory complication in pediatric HIV infection. The usual symptom is chronic cough. The chest radiograph reveals an interstitial nodular pattern. The diagnosis is made by persistent chest radiographic findings lasting more than 2 months without another documented cause. The course of the disease is variable, with waxing and waning of symptoms. Treatment with antiretrovirals and IV immunoglobulin may improve symptoms. Use of steroids for LIP is controversial.

The management of the child with acute pulmonary symptoms is given in Figure 6–1. As in adults, the most

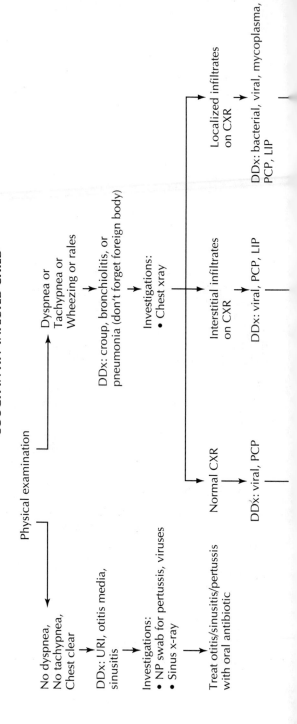

COUGH IN HIV-INFECTED CHILD

Physical examination

No dyspnea,
No tachypnea,
Chest clear

DDx: URI, otitis media,
sinusitis

Investigations:
• NP swab for pertussis, viruses
• Sinus x-ray

Treat otitis/sinusitis/pertussis
with oral antibiotic

Dyspnea or
Tachypnea or
Wheezing or rales

DDx: croup, bronchiolitis, or
pneumonia (don't forget foreign body)

Investigations:
• Chest xray

Normal CXR

DDx: viral, PCP

Interstitial infiltrates
on CXR

DDx: viral, PCP, LIP

Localized infiltrates
on CXR

DDx: bacterial, viral, mycoplasma,
PCP, LIP

If mild respiratory distress:
• ensure PCP prophylaxis if indicated. FU in 24 hrs.

If mod–severe respiratory distress:
• Admit, manage for respiratory symptoms (blood gases, oxygen, etc.), treat for PCP.
• Repeat CXR in 24 hrs.

If mild respiratory distress:
• Investigate by NP swab for pertussis and viruses, sputum if possible. Alternatives: induced sputum or auger suction or BAL.
• Treat for PCP.

If mod–severe respiratory distress:
• Admit, manage for respiratory symptoms (blood gases, oxygen, etc.), treat for PCP.
• Investigate: sputum if possible, BAL.

If mild respiratory distress:
• Investigate by NP swab for pertussis and viruses, sputum if possible: induced sputum or auger suction or BAL.
• Treat for bacteria ± mycoplasma.
• Ensure PCP prophylaxis is adequate.

If mod–severe respiratory distress:
• Admit, manage for respiratory symptoms (blood gases, oxygen, etc.), treat for PCP.
• Investigate: sputum if possible, BAL, and blood culture.
• Treat for bacterial pneumonia, PCP ± mycoplasma.

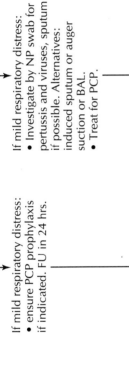

FIGURE 6–1

Management of Cough in the HIV-Infected Child. *Comments:* LIP is very common, but in an acutely ill child, it is a diagnosis of exclusion. Management of tuberculosis is indicated if there is a risk factor by history.

TABLE 6-2

Drug Dosages for Drugs Commonly Used in Children with HIV Infections

Antiretroviral Agents	
Zidovudine (AZT)	90–180 mg/m^2/dose QID
Didanosine (ddI)	60 mg/m^2/dose TID or 90 mg/m^2/dose BID
Zalcitabine (ddC)	0.005–0.01 mg/kg/dose TID
Lamivudine (3TC)	4 mg/kg/dose BID

Prophylaxis for Opportunistic Infections	
Pneumocystis carinii Pneumonia	
TMP-SMX	2.5 mg/kg/dose TMP BID daily or 3 days/week
Pentamidine	IV: 4 mg/kg/dose q 2–4 weeks Aerosolized by Respigard II inhaler: 300 mg/month
Dapsone	1–2 mg/kg/dose once daily
Toxoplasmosis	
Pyrimethamine	1–2 mg/kg/dose once daily
Sulfadiazine	25–100 mg/kg/dose once daily
Candida	
Ketoconazole	5–10 mg/kg/dose once or twice daily
Fluconazole	3–6 mg/kg/dose once daily
Itraconazole	2–5 mg/kg/dose once daily
Mycobacterium Avium Complex	
Rifabutin	300 mg once daily for children >6 years 5 mg/kg/day for children <6 years
Herpes Simplex (suppression)	
Acyclovir	PO: 10 mg/kg/dose BID (max 400 mg/dose)

common opportunistic infection is PCP. The highest risk period for infection is during infancy, from 2 to 8 months of age. The CD4 count is not as useful as in adults as an indicator of risk of PCP. Any one of the following are indications for PCP prophylaxis:

- Indeterminate HIV status from 1 month of age until status established.

- Previous PCP.

- Symptomatic HIV disease.

- CD4 count <500 for age 1 to 5 years, <200 for age ≥6 years.

The drugs and dosages for pediatric PCP prophylaxis are given in Table 6–2. The agents used are the same as for adults. Aerosolized pentamidine is not practical for younger children (<7 years), who have difficulty using inhalers; therefore IV pentamidine is usually preferable in these patients. Older children may receive aerosolized pentamidine using the Respigard II as for adults.

GASTROINTESTINAL MANIFESTATIONS

Diarrhea is the most common GI symptom in HIV-infected children. A viral etiology is common, although the pathogens listed for adults can also be pathogenic in children. Adequate hydration should be ensured but withholding of food longer than 24 hours is to be avoided. For infants with prolonged diarrhea the use of a lactose-free milk-based or soy formula should be considered.

CENTRAL NERVOUS SYSTEM MANIFESTATIONS

Central nervous system (CNS) symptoms may be the first HIV-associated problems to develop in an infant and may occur despite normal CD4 counts. These symptoms include the following:

- Cognitive delays.
- Memory deficits.
- Behavioral problems.
- Growth delays.
- Motor disabilities.
- Loss of developmental milestones.

The approach to acute or focal neurologic changes should be as for adults because the same CNS opportunistic infections can occur in children, but are less common than in adults.

References

1. Mofenson LM. Epidemiology and determinants of vertical HIV transmission. Semin Pediatr Infect Dis 1994; 5:252–65.
2. Connor EM, Sperling RS, Gelber R, et al. Reduction of maternal–infant transmission of human immundeficiency virus type I with zidovudine treatment. N Engl J Med 1994; 331: 1173–80.
3. Centers for Disease Control and Prevention. 1994 Revised classification system for human immunodeficiency virus infection in children less than 13 years of age. MMWR 1994; 43(RR-12): 1–10.
4. National Working Group, Health Canada. A comprehensive

guide for the care of persons with HIV disease. Module 2: Infants, children and youth. The College of Family Physicians of Canada, 1995.

5. Working Group on Antiretroviral Therapy: National Pediatric HIV Resource Center. Antiretroviral therapy and medical management of the human immunodeficiency virus-infected child. Pediatr Infect Dis J 1993; 12:513–22.

7

The Role of Nursing in HIV/ AIDS Care

Georgina Veldhorst, R.N., M.Sc.

Joyce Fenuta, R.N.

Helen Harrison, R.N.

THE CHANGING ROLE OF THE NURSE

In general patient care, nursing continues to evolve from a medical approach to illness into a more holistic health care model. The evolving role of the professional nurse has been limited by the restrictive nature of institutional structures, policies, and procedures and by the focus on task completion. A result of these restrictions has been that practices that fail to meet the needs of the patient are often left unchallenged as care is frequently not individualized to the specific patient. Providing care to people with HIV/AIDS offers an excellent opportunity for nurses to implement new models of care.

Changing accountability, along with a partnering relationship between the nurse and patient, creates a clear picture of the need for coordination, advocacy, and facilitation by the nurse on behalf of the patient. The professional nurse attempts to develop therapeutic relationships built on goals that are patient driven and mutually established. Patient-centered plans incorporate the actual response of the individual and allow for patients to have control of their health care. Nurses are responsible for meeting practice standards, developing therapeutic relationships, and setting mutual care plans. Although nurses have traditionally coordinated care, they are now able to establish and maintain the coordinator role, as their accountability is clear, and new lines of communication among the patient, significant others, and agencies are established.

Many nurses and patients believe that the nurse could be

the most effective coordinator of patient care. This coordi-nation of care has often been done on an informal level, as structures or positions such as the "charge nurse," have filtered the communication from the staff nurse to other health care providers, both within and outside of the organization. The many demands on a nurse's time, the heavy focus on tasks, the emphasis on the patient's immediate needs, and the lack of continuity of the nurse care giver has limited the formalization of this coordinator role.

Plans of care are tools that nurses have at their disposal, but are frequently not fully valued or used appropriately. Nursing care plans often utilize standardized plans into which the patient's diagnosis best fits, not reflecting the individual human response to illness. Maintaining these plans at times is seen as another task that needs to be completed, and not as a potentially effective method of communication for the improvement of patient care. The nurse, in practice, is in a position to develop a unique relationship with the patient, gaining insight into the individual's needs, but does not validate this assessment with the patient or communicate these findings with other care providers in a formal way. This creates further barriers to effective communication between the patient and the health care team.

NURSING IN HIV/AIDS CARE

People with HIV/AIDS have frequent interactions with the health care system throughout the course of their HIV infection. HIV has complex physical manifestations affect-ing the body, mind, and spirit of the individual. In most areas of the world, including many communities within North America, an extensive team of health care experts, from diverse professional groups, are not readily available to provide a wide range of expertise. In most settings nurses and physicians collaborate with the HIV-infected patient to optimize health. In order to maximize patient outcomes cost effectively nurses must work from a different paradigm.

Throughout the course of the infection, an individual is likely to use many, if not all of the following health care settings: primary, home, day, acute, respite, chronic, and palliative care, and bereavement follow-up. In order for nurses to be able to provide the services that patients want or need, continuity of care and the care giver should be established across the continuum from primary care through to palliative care. This continuity would benefit the patient, as a core group of providers know the patient's story well. To be most effective the same nurse should coordinate care across as much of the continuum as his or her expertise allows. Where provision of nursing care is not possible by the same nurse, comprehensive effective communication with other providers is essential. What the patient values, what his or her wishes are, who is aware of the patient's diagnosis, and what advanced directives are in place are pieces of the story the nurse should know and share with the patient's permission. The care plan is an excellent tool to communicate important information to other providers, particularly when the patient needs emergency or inpatient care. To facilitate empowering the patient and increasing the effectiveness of communication, the patient may be encouraged to bring an updated copy of the plan of care to all interactions with the health care system. In order for the patient to be served well, nurses need to move away from the typical focus on tasks seen in many hospitals and other settings and toward the establishment of a long-range continuous professional relationship with the patient and their significant others.

CARE PLANNING

The patient care plan is a communication mechanism, developed and utilized by a nurse and a patient to convey information about the individual patient to other nurses and members of the interdisciplinary care team. The care plan, when properly developed, gives control of health and the healing process to the patient.[1]

Plan Development

The nursing process (assessment, diagnosis, planning, implementation, and evaluation) is the framework utilized by the nurse in care plan development. The coordinating nurse uses assessment skills to gain a comprehensive understanding of the patient's unique life experiences/ situation, feelings, behaviors, perceptions, values, and physical manifestations and uses this information to formulate individualized plans of care with the patient.

Knowing the patient is central to the nurse–patient relationship. To know the patient means to appreciate the patient's typical pattern of response and to know "the person." This way of "knowing" is central to skilled clinical judgment. It is the prerequisite for all planning, implementation of intervention, and evaluation of outcomes. "Knowing" the patient sets up the opportunity for patient advocacy.[2]

The plan of care includes both short- and long-term goals that are unique to the individual. Determining these goals may require the nurse and other team members to provide objective information on treatment options. The patient should be able to expect the knowledge and expertise of the nurse to be integrated with the patient's values and beliefs. The goals, plans, and interventions should be developed with the patient and must be documented in a manner acceptable to the patient. Quality of life is defined by the patient; the individual identifies those qualities that will ensure a meaningful existence. The health care team should be prepared to support the patient's preference.

It is essential that the patient has input into and is in agreement with all aspects of the plan in order for this plan to be meaningful. Just as planning of care is done mutually with the patient, evaluation of the outcomes of care should be done collaboratively with the patient.

Planning for the future needs of the patient should be an integral part of providing care for a person living with HIV/AIDS. This should include adequate support in the home, assistive devices, discharge from acute care settings, palliative care, funeral arrangements, and bereavement follow-up.

PLAN UTILIZATION

The coordinating nurse uses the plan of care to facilitate continuity of care through communication with other nurses and members of the care team. Care is coordinated within and between the primary, home, day, acute, chronic, and palliative care settings, with an emphasis on effective communication between the providers at the various settings.

It is essential that all interdisciplinary members be aware of the patient's specific goals as identified during plan development. Patient care conferences provide an opportunity to review the patient goals. The coordinating nurse would present the "patient's story" for discussion with the care team. Multiprofessional collaboration is important when plans are revised, providing a broader perspective of the patient's situation. Nurses are responsible for continually collaborating with their patients to update and discuss progress toward these goals. Most importantly, the person receiving care should be able to expect that health care will be coordinated and delivered in partnership with him or her.

People with HIV/AIDS could benefit significantly from the role of the nurse as coordinator providing continuity of care. The coordinating nurse would utilize the plan of care developed in partnership with the patient to ensure effective communication of the patient's needs and wishes with the other care providers. Although nurses have traditionally coordinated care, they are now able to establish and maintain the coordinator role, as accountability is clear, and lines of communication are established between the patient, significant others, and agencies.

References

1. Wesorick B. Standards of Nursing Care: A Model for Clinical Practice. Philadelphia: JB Lippincott, 1990.
2. Tanner C, Benner P, Chesla C, Gordon D. The phenomenology of knowing the patient. Image: J Nurs Scholarship 1993; 25(4).

System- and Problem-Oriented Evaluation

RESPIRATORY MANIFESTATIONS

Charles K. N. Chan M.D., F.R.C.P.C., F.C.C.P., F.A.C.P.

Although HIV compromises principally the cellular immune arm of the host defense system, bacterial respiratory tract infection has been recognized as a frequent and potentially severe problem in HIV patients. The infecting bacterial pathogens resemble those in non-HIV patients and include *Pneumococcus* and *Haemophilus influenzae,* and in recent years *Pseudomonas species* has been identified as another significant respiratory pathogen as well.

Opportunistic infections affecting the respiratory system generally do not pose a problem until the CD4 count falls below 200 or when the percentage of CD4 drops below 15 percent. Despite effective prophylaxis, *Pneumocystis carinii* pneumonia (PCP) remains the most common opportunistic infection in AIDS patients. *Mycobacterium tuberculosis* has also become more frequent, and in certain endemic regions, fungal infections, including *Cryptococcus* and *Histoplasma,* are also quite prevalent.

Atypical *Mycobacterium avium-intracellulare* (MAI), or *Mycobacterium avium* complex (MAC), is another contributing pathogen but in distinction to the other respiratory pathogens, tends to present as a multisystem infective process rather than just in the respiratory tract.

The following outlines the basic steps that may help in the initial assessment and management of respiratory problems in HIV-infected patients. These steps are particularly useful for Emergency Department and urgent outpatient assessment of HIV-infected individuals with cough and dyspnea.

DIAGNOSTIC STEPS

Step I: Background Information

Most HIV-infected patients are well aware of their most recent CD4 count and whether or not opportunistic infection is likely. Patients already on PCP prophylaxis or some other form of antiretroviral, such as zidovudine (AZT), didanosine (ddI), zalcitabine (ddC), or lamivudine (3TC), would also suggest they likely have low CD4 counts (<200 to 300), and thus are at risk of developing opportunistic infections. Furthermore, any patient with a previous episode of PCP has advanced immunosuppression.

Step II: Stratification According to Clinical Presentation

The first step is to take a history and do a physical examination in order to classify the presenting respiratory ailment as having an infectious or a noninfectious etiology. Where infection is suspected, one should attempt to differentiate between bacterial and nonbacterial etiologies.

The clinical presentation of bacterial infections in a patient with HIV is very similar to that in non-HIV patients, that is, fever, cough productive of mucopurulent sputum with or without blood, and increased dyspnea. The only exception in HIV subjects is that the illness might have gone on for several days up to a week, rather than for a shorter period, and the patients may look less "toxic."

Nonbacterial respiratory infection and noninfectious respiratory complications have very similar presentations. The patients are usually ill for some time, ranging from weeks to months, often with a nonproductive cough, dyspnea, sporadic low-grade fever, sweats, fatigue, malaise, and weight loss.

Step III: Stratification According to Routine Laboratory Tests

Routine laboratory tests on HIV patients with acute respiratory difficulties should include a CBC, chest x-ray, and serum LDH determination.

White blood cell (WBC) count in HIV patients with advanced immunosuppression is typically low (2000 to 3000 range). Thus, a WBC in the 7000 to 9000 range should raise some concerns about either a primary bacterial or a concurrent bacterial infectious process. On the other hand, nonbacterial and noninfectious complications would typically show a WBC in the 2000 to 3000 range. Lymphopenia is seen in all HIV patients, and is usually not helpful in the diagnostic decision-making process. Serum LDH is by no means specific for PCP, but a substantial elevation in LDH in the absence of liver function test abnormalities, normal muscles enzymes, and little evidence of hemolysis is strongly indicative of PCP.

A chest x-ray is helpful because bacterial complications often present with focal findings such as lobar pneumonia and at times multifocal segmental distribution, whereas nonbacterial complications range from hilar adenopathy to pleural effusions to diffuse interstitial infiltrates. A summary of likely diagnoses based on chest radiographic findings is shown in Table 8–1. Patients who have been on PCP prophylaxis, such as aerosol pentamidine, tend to have upper lung zone distribution with a PCP relapse. It should also be noted that upper lobe infiltrates have been described in early PCP relapse in HIV patients on systemic prophylaxis including dapsone.

Step IV: Specific Diagnostic Tests

Routine blood cultures and MAC blood cultures are advised. Sputum should be sent for regular Gram stain, acid fast bacilli (AFB) stain, and direct fluorescent antibody (DFA) stain for PCP. For those patients who appear to have bacterial infection, suggested by the chest x-ray and routine laboratory tests, one can probably stop the investigation at this point and start patients on empiric therapy pending culture results.

For patients whose findings are most consistent with PCP, specific therapy is advised and the only remaining question is whether further diagnostic tests are required. A sputum or induced sputum stain positive for PCP provides confirmation. On the other hand, if the sputum gives no clues, bronchoscopy would be the next logical investigation. For those patients who have not had PCP previously, it is probably best, at least for the first episode, to obtain definitive proof. For those who have had more than one bout of PCP, the only time bronchoscopy is essential is when the patient has multiple drug allergies and requires salvage or

TABLE 8-1

Classification of HIV-Related Pulmonary Diseases Based on Chest Radiographic Features

Focal (Segmental or Single Lobe) Interstitial/Alveolar Process

Bacterial (including *Mycoplasma/Chlamydia/Legionella*)
Fungi
Mycobacteria
Actinomycosis
Nocardia
Pneumocystis
Lymphoma

Diffuse (Multilobar) Interstitial/Alveolar Process

Pneumocystis
Bacterial (including *Mycoplasma/Chlamydia/Legionella*)
Lymphocytic interstitial pneumonitis
Kaposi's sarcoma
Mycobacteria
Fungi
Viruses (including herpes and CMV)
Bronchiolitis obliterans organizing pneumonia (BOOP)

Hilar Adenopathy

Lymphoma
Mycobacteria
Fungi
Kaposi's sarcoma

Pleural Effusion(s) +/− Masses

Empyema
Kaposi's sarcoma
Lymphoma
Mycobacteria

Multiple Nodular Lesions

Kaposi's sarcoma
Mycobacteria
Fungi
Viruses (including herpes and CMV)

experimental anti-PCP medications. If the illness does not respond to treatment, bronchoscopy should be done to confirm PCP or detect another condition. Concerns about drug toxicity may interrupt treatment and call for definitive proof about the advisability of switching from one drug combination to another. Most patients whose clinical and radiologic pictures are compatible with PCP can be treated empirically. If bronchoscopy is to be carried out, it can be done within a week of starting treatment with a yield that is still quite high.

If there is no confirmation of either bacterial or PCP, bronchoscopy and other investigations are usually necessary, especially if there are no AFB on sputum smear. If AFB are found in sputum, other investigations, including bronchoscopy, should be initiated and the patient should be placed in respiratory isolation (see the discussion of tuberculosis in the Opportunistic Injections section later in this chapter). Early in an episode of PCP, the chest x-ray may still be normal. Pulmonary function tests (diffusing capacity) and a gallium lung scan may indicate impairment or abnormality in lung fields and justify further invasive procedures such as bronchoscopy.

Although there has been some concern about the yield of bronchoscopy and bronchoalveolar lavage (BAL) for the diagnosis of PCP in the era of routine prophylaxis, which may reduce the load of *Pneumocystis* organisms in the yield, the utilization of more sensitive staining methods, including DFA stain, has generally obviated the need to go on to transbronchial lung biopsy in the majority of the patients. Newer and more sensitive tools, such as the polymerase chain reaction (PCR) technique for *Pneumocystis,* should further enhance our diagnostic accuracy using BAL sampling.

Step V: Assessment for Needs for Admission to Hospital

Medical Assessment

The general status of the patient determines the need for hospitalization. Patients should be admitted if they have difficulty eating or drinking, have fluctuating levels of consciousness, and most certainly if they are severely dehydrated. Assessment of oxygenation is essential and can be done by oximetry. If the patient's oxygen saturation is less than 90 percent, even before therapy, they are likely to get worse and should be hospitalized. If an arterial blood gas level is obtained and is below 60 mm Hg, the patient should be admitted.

Most patients can then be discharged and started on PO therapy. However, those who are sick enough to be admitted should probably be started on IV therapy, especially if they have difficulty eating and drinking, and then be switched to PO therapy once they stabilize.

Psychosocial Assessment

Not infrequently, although the patient's condition may seem satisfactory, admission may still be desirable because of psychosocial situations. Lack of support at home, inability to care for oneself, and fear of death from AIDS are some of the frequently encountered circumstances that might benefit from a short-term stabilization. The objective of the admission is to provide support and reassurance, and to allow the patient to regain confidence that treatment being implemented is going well and recovery is well on its way.

Step VI: Follow-up Arrangement and Advice to the Patient upon Discharge from the Emergency Department

When discharged from the Emergency Department, therapy may be started at once for bacterial, PCP, and other nonbacterial respiratory complications, but the patient must be urged to see his or her own HIV family practitioner(s) as soon as possible. Patients should also be told to return to the Emergency Department if their symptoms remain or worsen despite treatment. If there is any doubt about a patient's ability to obtain appropriate follow-up and investigation, arrangement should be made with the local institutional HIV/Infectious Disease or pulmonary consult service(s) for follow-up investigation and monitoring of treatment.

THERAPEUTICS

Bacterial Pneumonia

Because of their impaired immune system, HIV patients should be treated for 10 to 14 days, as their response to therapy is typically slower than that of immunocompetent subjects.

The first decision regarding selection of antibiotics for bacterial pneumonia while culture results are pending is whether one needs to cover for *Pseudomonas*. Patients at risk for *Pseudomonas* infection include patients who have had repeated courses of antibiotics, prior bronchiectasis, recent courses of corticosteroids, or recent hospitalizations.

The second therapeutic decision is whether coverage for atypical pathogens (*Mycoplasma, Chlamydia, Legionella*) is necessary. The newer macrolides/azalides can cover both the usual bacterial pathogens and the atypical pathogens, but if

TABLE 8-2

Empiric Antimicrobial Suggestions for HIV Patients with Suspected Pneumonia*

Bacterial (non-Pseudomonas)	
Amoxicillin/clavunate	500 mg PO TID
TMP-SMX	2 DS PO BID
Clarithromycin	500 mg PO BID
Cefuroxime axetil	500 mg PO BID
Cefaclor	500 mg PO TID
Bacterial (Pseudomonas)	
Ciprofloxacin†	500 mg PO BID
Ofloxacin†	400 mg PO BID
Mycoplasma/Chlamydia/Legionella	
Clarithromycin	500 mg PO BID
Azithromycin	500 mg PO daily

*For the treatment of PCP, refer to the discussion of PCP later in this chapter.

†Additional coverage for Streptococcus may be necessary.

adequacy of coverage is in doubt, double agents should be used.

Table 8–2 includes some of the more popular antimicrobial agents and the recommended dosages.

Pneumocystis Carinii Pneumonia

For the current therapeutic options in the treatment of PCP, refer to the discussion of PCP in the Opportunistic Infections section, later in this chapter.

To date, trimethoprim-sulfamethoxazole (TMP-SMX) resistance is still difficult to determine. However, based on available clinical data, TMP-SMX remains the first-line treatment option for PCP. For patients who are intolerant of TMP-SMX, up to half of the subjects can tolerate the combination of dapsone plus trimethoprim. Other systemic treatment options and dosages are included in the discussion of PCP.

Suggested Readings

ATS official statement: Fungal infection in HIV-infected persons. Am J Respir Crit Care Med 1995; 152: 816–22.

McGuinness G, Scholes JV, Garray SM, et al. Cytomegalovirus pneumonitis: Spectrum of parenchymal CT findings with pathologic correlation in 21 AIDS patients. Radiology 1994; 192: 451–9.

Murray JF, Mills J. Pulmonary infectious complications of human immunodeficiency virus infection. Part I. Am Rev Respir Dis 1990; 141: 1356–72.

Murray JF, Mills J. Pulmonary infectious complications of human immunodeficiency virus infection. Part II. Am Rev Respir Dis 1990; 141: 1582–98.

White DA, Matthay RA. Noninfectious pulmonary complications of infection with the human immunodeficiency virus. Am Rev Respir Dis 1989; 140: 1763–87.

GASTROINTESTINAL MANIFESTATIONS

Gabor Kandel, M.D., F.R.C.P.C.

ABDOMINAL PAIN

General Issues

Abdominal pain in the AIDS patient is often due to non-HIV-related diseases, unlike other symptoms such as dyspnea and diarrhea, which almost invariably are related in some way to HIV infection. An unusually wide variety of conditions can cause abdominal pain. Therefore, if possible, the differential diagnosis should revolve around an associated abnormality, such as diarrhea or elevated serum alkaline phosphatase, rather than around the pain itself.

Symptom Clusters and Investigations

The approach to abdominal pain, including indications for investigations and surgery, is not significantly different from that in non-HIV-infected patients. The chief exception is that HIV patients with abdominal pain have an unusually high incidence of hepatobiliary disease. For example, sclerosing cholangitis, which has been well described in AIDS, is characterized by gradually progressive abdominal pain, most often in the right upper quadrant or epigastrium, elevated serum alkaline phosphatase, and hepatomegaly. Jaundice is rare, whereas in the cholangitis seen in immunocompetent hosts, it is a common finding. Dilated and thickened biliary ducts (extrahepatic, intrahepatic, or both) can usually be seen upon abdominal ultrasonography and/or computed tomography (CT), but a definitive diagnosis requires endoscopic retrograde cholangiopancreatography (ERCP) to demonstrate the strictures and focal dilations in the biliary tree. Pathogenesis is unclear: some reports have implicated infection by cytomegalovirus (CMV), often with concomitant *Cryptosporidium* or *Microsporidium* infection. Satisfactory treatment is not available. However, endoscopic sphincterotomy has been described as beneficial if the common bile duct is dilated to the level of the ampulla of Vater, suggestive of papillary stenosis.

Acalculous cholecystitis is also more common in the AIDS population, and is most frequently due to CMV and/or *Cryptosporidium* infection. Diagnosis is based on a combination of four characteristic features: (1) acute, constant pain in the right upper quadrant or epigastrium, (2) fever, (3) dilation and edema of the gallbladder on ultrasonography (or CT scan), and (4) the absence of uptake of isotope into the gallbladder on a hepatic iminodiacetic acid (HIDA) scan. Antibiotics are almost never helpful. Cholecystectomy is curative, but it is often difficult to know whether or not to recommend this operation if not all of the above-described features are present. It is common, for example, to see HIV-infected patients with upper-abdominal pain and a thick-walled gallbladder but a normal HIDA scan (i.e., the normal isotope uptake is seen in the gallbladder). Moreover, fever can often be attributed to other diseases, such as disseminated *Mycobacterium avium* complex (MAC) infection, which may not be the cause of the abdominal pain. In this situation, "watchful waiting" is indicated, with a view toward surgery only if there is no improvement with time and analgesics. The septic shock and dramatic clinical deterioration classically described in calculous cholecystitis allowed to progress without surgical intervention is almost never seen in HIV-related acalculous cholecystitis.

Lymphoma characteristically presents with abdominal pain, since the gastrointestinal tract, especially the stomach, is the most common extranodal organ involved by this disease. In obscure cases of pain, there is often a worry that lymphoma is being missed. However, lymphoma in the setting of HIV infection is usually disseminated by the time of presentation, so that the diagnosis is almost always suggested clinically, or with a test such as abdominal ultrasonography/CT, endoscopy, or barium studies of the gastrointestinal tract. The diagnosis is then established by either endoscopic biopsy of the bowel or percutaneous biopsy of the liver.

Intestinal diseases usually cause diarrhea, and not isolated abdominal pain, but sometimes colitis or enteritis from pathogens such as CMV and *Clostridium difficile* are not associated with a change in bowel habits. A useful clue to this condition is exacerbation of the pain with eating, and relief after defecation. Toxic megacolon and colonic perforations have been described in the absence of diarrhea and rectal bleeding; in AIDS this is more often due to infections than idiopathic inflammatory bowel disease (as in non-HIV patients). Kaposi's sarcoma is relatively common in the bowel, but it only rarely causes symptoms other than gastrointestinal bleeding.

Other causes of abdominal pain in HIV include pancreatitis, caused by drugs such as didanosine (ddI) or pentamidine or by alcoholism, which is more common in HIV patients than the general population. Diagnosis can be difficult because an elevation in serum amylase is often due in AIDS to "macroamylasemia" (a benign condition characterized by clustering of amylase molecules that cannot be readily filtered by the kidney because of their high molecular weight).

Ascites can also present with abdominal pain and bloating, secondary to liver disease (especially chronic hepatitis B). An idiopathic high-protein ("exudative") ascites has been described in AIDS patients without features of portal hypertension or hepatic dysfunction.

HIV-related causes of acute "surgical" abdominal pain with peritonitis include perforated bowel from CMV infection, Kaposi's sarcoma, and lymphoma. These conditions can also cause intestinal obstruction. Mycobacterial peritonitis and intussusception from mass lesions have also been described. Surgery is indicated in peritonitis, just as in non-HIV-infected patients.

Dyspepsia, nausea, and vomiting are most frequently due to medications. Peptic ulcer is uncommon if the CD4 cell count is low, since most such patients produce little gastric acid. Empiric histamine H_2 therapy is therefore only rarely recommended, unlike in non-HIV-infected individuals.

DIARRHEA

Clinical Evaluation

Prospective studies have demonstrated that at least 50 percent of patients with HIV infection will suffer at some point in their illness from diarrhea, as defined by a change in stool consistency or frequency. This not only is a disabling symptom, but often contributes to weight loss, a chief underlying cause of death in AIDS.

Large-volume watery movements accompanied by malabsorption, bloating, and cramps are said to indicate that the small bowel is diseased, whereas frequent, small-volume, painful movements associated with tenesmus, mucoid stools, and rectal bleeding point toward large-bowel conditions. However, it should be emphasized that no studies are available to determine whether a history focusing on these features has any value in determining the cause of diarrhea in HIV infection.

On the other hand, certain questions are clearly critical. For example, the length of time diarrhea has been present should be determined, since acute diarrhea tends to be caused more often by bacteria than chronic symptoms. Weight loss indicates the severity of the disease underlying the diarrhea, and determines the need for nutritional support (see under Treatment). CD4 count is important, since the spectrum of pathogens causing diarrhea, and the efficacy of treatment, are determined by this marker of immunosuppression (Table 8–3). Other important features of the history include

TABLE 8–3

Absolute CD4 Count as a Predictor of Potential Pathogens Causing Diarrheal Disease*

PATHOGEN	ABSOLUTE CD4 COUNT ($\times 10^6$/L)	
	>200†	<100
Bacteria	Salmonella Shigella Campylobacter Yersinia Clostridium difficile Mycobacterium tuberculosis	Escherichia coli Mycobacterium avium
Viruses	Adenovirus Rotavirus Herpes simplex virus ?HIV	Cytomegalovirus
Protoza	Giardia lamblia Entamoeba histolytica	Microsporidium Cryptosporidium‡ Isospora Cyclospora

*Guidelines only; exceptions may be observed.

†All of the pathogens listed in this column may be seen in more immunocompromised patients as well.

‡Causes chronic diarrhea in this group only, but can precipitate a self-limited illness in more immunocompetent patients (CD4 >180).

(Modified from Mayer and Wanke, 1994.)

exposure to antibiotics, local outbreaks of diarrhea, ingestion of unusual foods, and travel to other countries.

Extent of fluid loss can be judged by blood pressure, pulse (and positional changes in these parameters), jugular venous pressure, and skin turgor. Other findings worth specifically seeking include organomegaly (as a clue to lymphoma), skin rashes (as a clue to vitamin deficiencies secondary to malabsorption), and retinal disease (as a clue to CMV infection).

Investigations

A consensus has emerged that investigations should start with stool analysis. At least three stool specimens are examined with saline, iodine, modified acid-fast stain (or immunofluorescence) for *Cryptosporidium,* and a trichome (or chitin) stain for *Microsporidium.* Stool should also be sent for culture (including *Clostridium difficile*) and *C. difficile* toxin. Blood cultures for MAC and salmonellae are appropriate if the patient is febrile: in AIDS these organisms can be absent in stool yet isolated from blood (Table 8–4). The clinical significance of MAC isolated only from stool is unclear, but this probably represents carriage rather than true infection.

If no pathogens are found, and if the diarrhea persists, stool analysis should be repeated. In at least one series of patients, this had a higher yield than endoscopy.

Necessary blood tests include serum creatinine, electrolytes, complete blood cell count, albumin, and liver en-

TABLE 8–4

Gastrointestinal Pathogens in HIV-Infected Patients

ORGAN	PATHOGENS
Stomach	Cytomegalovirus; *Mycobacterium avium-intracellulare*
Small intestine	*Cryptosporidium; Microsporidium; Isospora belli; Mycobacterium avium-intracellular; Salmonella* species; *Campylobacter jejuni*
Colon	Cytomegalovirus; *Cryptosporidium; Mycobacterium avium-intracellulare; Shigella flexneri; Clostridium difficile; Campylobacter jejuni; Histoplasma capsulatum;* adenovirus; herpes simplex virus (rectum)

zymes. Anemia, neutropenia, and elevated serum alkaline phosphatase are useful clues to disseminated MAC infection.

From this point on, the value of further investigations is controversial. Endoscopy can detect pathogens not found by stool analysis, but the risk/morbidity to benefit ratio of these invasive tests is unclear. For example, one review has suggested that the yield of complete evaluation is so low as to be not worthwhile if the diarrhea responds to symptomatic therapy with loperamide (Imodium). On the other hand, this approach has been questioned since endoscopy can detect treatable pathogens, albeit only in about 20 percent of cases. Accordingly, if the patient agrees to an aggressive diagnostic approach, endoscopy should be offered, starting with colonoscopy if the diarrhea pattern suggests colonic disease, followed by duodenal biopsy provided no pathogens are found. Alternatively, if small-bowel infection is suggested clinically, duodenal biopsy is done before colonoscopy. Mucosal biopsies obtained at the time of endoscopy should be sent for hematoxylin and eosin (H&E) histology, virology, and mycobacteria culture. Patients should be warned before recommending endoscopy that "idiopathic" diarrhea is common in AIDS.

The major pathogen found by colonoscopy is CMV. Initial experience suggested that sigmoidoscopy was sufficient to detect the virus in most cases, but more recent reviews have shown that this pathogen is found exclusively in the right colon in about 40 percent of patients. The diagnosis is most clearly established if four criteria are met: mucosal colonic ulcers at endoscopy, CMV effect on H&E stain, CMV on in situ hybridization (or immunofluorescence), and isolation of the virus from the mucosal biopsy. Isolation of the virus from the biopsy, without the other three features, may represent contamination of the specimen by blood, and therefore is not by itself diagnostic. In one study, 25 percent of cases had normal endoscopic findings, but had all the other three diagnostic features.

Organisms detectable by duodenal biopsy, but easily missed on stool microscopy, include microsporidia, cryptosporidia, *Giardia,* and MAC.

Treatment of Specific Pathogens

Recommended therapeutic regimens are listed in Table 8–5. Many of the drugs eradicate pathogens only when the CD4 count is >200.

TABLE 8-5

Treatment of Bowel Infections

AGENT OF INFECTION	ANTIBIOTIC(S)	DURATION
Campylobacter sp.	Erythromycin 500 mg q6h PO	10–14 days
Salmonella sp.	Ciprofloxacin 500 mg BID PO	10–14 days, then maintenance
Shigella sp.	Based on susceptibility (virtually all isolates susceptible to ciprofloxacin) 500 mg BID	10–14 days (initial)
Entamoeba histolytica	Metronidazole 750 TID PO	10–14 days
	Iodoquinol 650 mg TID PO	21 days
Giardia lamblia	Metronidazole 500 mg q8h PO	10–14 days
Isospora belli	Cotrimoxazole 4 tablets QID PO	10–14 days (initial)
Strongyloides stercoralis	Thiabendazole 22 mg/kg BID PO	2 days
Cytomegalovirus	Gancyclovir (IV) 5 mg/kg BID or	14 days
	*Foscarnet (IV) 60 mg/kg q8h (infuse over 2 hours)	

(Continued)

TABLE 8–5

Treatment of Bowel Infections (Continued)

AGENT OF INFECTION	ANTIBIOTIC(S)	DURATION
Herpes simplex	Acyclovir 200 mg/kg 5×/day PO or 5 mg/kg q8h IV	10–14 days (initially)
Chlamydia trachomatis	Doxycycline 100 mg BID PO	10–14 days
Spirochetosis	Metronidazole 500 mg q8h PO	10–14 days
Cryptosporidium species	Paromomycin 500 mg QID PO	14 days
Microsporidium species	Albendazole 400 mg BID PO	Indefinitely
Mycobacterium avium complex	See elsewhere in this book	

Treatment for cryptosporidia, disseminated MAC, microsporidia, and salmonellae should probably be given indefinitely.

Most species of *Entamoeba* isolated from HIV patients are nonpathogenic. Even when the laboratory reports *Entamoeba histolytica* in the stool, the odds are that this is actually *Entamoeba dispar,* a species indistinguishable by clinical laboratory techniques from *E. histolytica,* but almost never invasive. Thus treatment for *Entamoeba* rarely helps the diarrhea, even though it eradicates the infection.

A randomized trial has demonstrated that ganciclovir therapy for CMV colitis improves the endoscopic appearance of the colon, diminishes fever and weight loss, and reduces the frequency of extracolonic CMV infection, but does not affect the diarrhea. The value of maintenance therapy is controversial.

Treatment If No Enteric Pathogen Is Found

The most useful agent for symptomatic control of diarrhea is loperamide, generally required at doses of 4 mg q4h regularly. When taken on a PRN basis, as advised by the drug manufacturer, the drug is usually less effective. Side effects include abdominal cramps, but there is no realistic potential of CNS side-effects, tolerance, or addiction, despite the similarity of this drug's biochemical structure to narcotics. Diphenoxylate (Lomotil) is a satisfactory and sometimes more effective substitute for loperamide, but has a greater tendency to lead to addiction. Codeine and morphine usually add to loperamide's effect, although drowsiness and addiction tend to develop.

Zidovudine has been shown to improve enterocyte maturation and replication, both of which are decreased in HIV infection. This may help to increase body weight. An immune-boosting effect has also been described for this drug, which possibly helps to clear intestinal pathogens.

Dietary change is less helpful than most patients realize. A high-fiber diet supplemented by a psyllium seed preparation often increases stool consistency, thereby decreasing urgency and incontinence. However, stool volume is most often concomitantly increased and therefore only some patients benefit from this approach. Other advice that can be given to patients is listed in Table 8–6. Each tip is worth following only if symptomatic benefit results. Reducing calorie and protein intake often reduces stool output, but this goal should take second priority to maintaining weight and nutrition.

TABLE 8-6

Dietary Advice to Control Diarrhea

Avoid milk and dairy products.
Avoid caffeine (including carbonated beverages containing
  caffeine, chocolate, tea).
Try to drink and eat liquids and foods at room temperature
  (because substances at extreme temperatures precipitate
  bowel contractions).
Reduce fats (butter, fried foods, salad dressings, pastries).
Reduce fiber (bran, cereals, brown bread, raw fruits and
  vegetables, nuts).
Increase easily absorbed foods (rice, bananas, dry toast,
  applesauce, mashed potatoes).
Avoid highly gas-producing foods (beans, broccoli, cabbage,
  cauliflower, corn, cucumbers, beer, green peppers, brussels
  sprouts).

Octreotide (Sandostatin), a somatostatin analog, was
initially shown to decrease stool volume in a proportion of
AIDS patients with diarrhea when no pathogen was found.
If it is used, it should be started at a dose of 50 µg
subcutaneously, increasing the dose every 48 hours until the
maximum dose of 200 µg QID is reached. However, a recent
large placebo-controlled trial was not able to shown any
significant benefit from this drug. Of interest is that in this
study, placebo was associated with a decrease in stool
volume of about 25 percent, emphasizing the fluctuating
nature of "idiopathic" HIV-related diarrhea.

Indications for Admission

Extracellular fluid depletion and serum electrolyte abnormalities are best treated with IV fluids in hospital. Even when
repletion can be given by mouth, hospitalization is generally
necessary because such hypovolemia, hyponatremia, and
hypokalemia indicate that the diarrhea is severe.

HIV-related diarrhea without an identifiable infectious
pathogen characteristically fluctuates in intensity. When the
diarrhea is severe, often 48 to 72 hours of bed rest and IV
fluid are helpful; for unclear reasons, patients tend to feel
better for weeks after this form of therapy.

In hospital, an elemental diet can be tried, since it has been
described to both increase weight and decrease stool volume.
Unfortunately this diet is so unpalatable that it must be
administered by some form of tube feeding, either using the
nasogastric approach, or via a percutaneous feeding gastros-

tomy. Rarely, prolonged total bowel rest with parenteral nutrition is necessary.

ELEVATED LIVER ENZYMES
General Issues

Elevations in serum transaminases (alanine transaminase [ALT], aspartate transaminase [AST]) and/or liver alkaline phosphatase occur in over two-thirds of patients with AIDS. The clinical challenge is to determine if these biochemical abnormalities are (1) incidental findings (e.g., elevated ALT caused by pentamidine usually does not even require discontinuation of this drug), (2) clues to a multisystem opportunistic infection or tumor that is best diagnosed by investigations directed at tissues other than the liver (e.g., disseminated MAC infection causing elevated serum alkaline phosphatase is best diagnosed by blood culture), or (3) secondary to a hepatobiliary condition causing symptoms that requires tests aimed at the liver and biliary tree (e.g., sclerosing cholangitis leading to abdominal pain and elevated serum alkaline phosphatase). Hepatomegaly without changes in liver enzymes only rarely requires investigations, unless symptoms are present.

Symptom Clusters

A wide variety of conditions can involve the liver in HIV infection (Table 8–7). Once a liver enzyme is found to be elevated, the next step is to determine if the elevation is chiefly in transaminases or in alkaline phosphatase.

Treatable causes of significantly increased transaminases

TABLE 8–7
Causes of Liver Disease in AIDS

COMMON	UNCOMMON
Cytomegalovirus	Lymphoma*
Mycobacterium avium complex	Cryptococcus neoformans
Hepatitis B	Histoplasmosis capsulatum
Sclerosing cholangitis	Mycobacterium tuberculosis
Kaposi's sarcoma	Unspecified acid-fast bacilli
Steatosis	
Alcohol	

*Common in wide-spread disease, but rare in the absence of lymphoma elsewhere.

TABLE 8–8

Useful Blood Tests to Evaluate Elevated Liver Transaminases

HBsAg*
Anti-HCV (antibodies to hepatitis C)
Protein electrophoresis (although less useful than in non-HIV-
    infected patients)
Anti-HAV, IgM fraction
Serum iron, total iron-binding capacity, ferritin
Ceruloplasmin
Antinuclear factor, anti-smooth muscle antibodies
Alpha fetoprotein
Albumin
Prothrombin time/partial thromboplastin time
Platelet count
Bilirubin

Other markers of hepatitis B, such as anti-HBs and anti-HBc, can also be ordered, but only HBsAg indicates that the hepatitis B virus is causing the elevated liver enzymes. Antibodies to hepatitis B are simply markers of previous self-resolving infection; their presence or absence in the setting of elevated liver enzymes is not helpful. Anti-HDV (antibodies to the delta virus), HBeAg (hepatitis Be antigen), and anti-HBe should be measured in the serum if HBsAg is present.

can generally be found either by a history and physical examination or a battery of blood tests (Table 8–8). Emphasis should be placed on searching for hepatotoxic drugs (antituberculosis medications, trimethoprim-sulfamethoxazole, ketoconazole), past history of viral hepatitis, and alcohol abuse. Reviewing old medical records can be particularly rewarding. In the setting of elevated transaminases, fever without localizing symptoms points toward CMV hepatitis, a disease in which there are usually no complaints referable directly to the liver. Hepatitis B and alcoholic liver disease have an increased incidence in HIV-infected patients.

A predominantly elevated serum alkaline phosphatase also mandates a directed history and physical examination. Fever in this situation points toward disseminated MAC infection, especially if diarrhea and weight loss are also present. This infection is best diagnosed by culture of blood and, if necessary, by bone marrow examination. Sclerosing cholangitis, presumably secondary to infection of the bile ducts by *Cryptosporidium*, CMV and *Microsporidium* (alone or in combination), should be considered if abdominal pain is present.

Mass lesions, such as Kaposi's sarcoma, peliosis (from bacillary angiomatosis; particularly important to diagnose because it responds so well to antibiotics), lymphoma, and carcinoma, and infiltrating conditions, such as granulomas, also characteristically increase the alkaline phosphatase more than the transaminases.

Jaundice is uncommon, and is generally more indicative of the severity of liver disease rather than a clue to its cause.

Hepatotropic Viruses

At least 90 percent of HIV-infected patients have serologic evidence of hepatitis B infection, but this proportion is not significantly different from non-HIV-infected controls with risk factors for HIV. Hepatitis B does not increase mortality significantly in AIDS. Thus interferon is indicated only rarely, and less often leads to remission than in non-HIV-infected individuals. HIV has been described as altering hepatitis B infection in the following ways:

1. It increases the chance of chronicity after acute viral infection.

2. In chronic infection, it increases the chance that the virus will continue to replicate in the hepatocyte (i.e., it increases the proportion of patients with HBeAg, HBV DNA polymerase, HBV DNA in the serum).

3. It increases the risk of reactivation (i.e., spontaneous conversion from anti-HBe to HBeAg, or from anti-HBs to HBsAg; this transition is often associated with fulminant hepatic failure and death).

4. It *decreases* the extent of liver damage and transaminase elevation in chronic infection.

5. It decreases the chances of responding to the vaccine (although this should still be given if there is no serologic evidence of previous hepatitis B exposure).

6. It increases the rate of loss of anti-HBs from the serum.

Among HIV-infected patients, only IV drug users and hemophiliacs have a significantly higher incidence of hepatitis C than the general population. HIV has been described as accelerating the course of chronic hepatitis C, since cirrhosis has been described in this situation as developing within 3 years of exposure to the hepatitis C virus. Other reports, however, have not described this phenomenon. The rate of response of hepatitis C to interferon is not well described in HIV infection. The false-positive reactions obtained with the first-generation enzyme linked immunosorbent assay (ELISA) kits to detect anti-HCV are not a problem with the currently used tests.

Investigations

Abdominal ultrasonography should be considered in most patients with abnormal liver biochemistry, but is most useful if the alkaline phosphatase is elevated. In experienced hands, mass lesions are well seen. Biopsy is commonly necessary for a definitive diagnosis. Usually, a radiologically guided percutaneous aspiration with a fine needle is done first. If the cytology specimen obtained with this method is insufficient, a core should be obtained, either percutaneously (if the lesion is amenable to this approach, and in the absence of a bleeding tendency) or via laparoscopy.

Similarly, bile duct and/or gall bladder abnormalities are suggested on ultrasonography in most patients with "sclerosing cholangitis," but ERCP is necessary for a definitive diagnosis. The pain caused by this condition has been described as being relieved by endoscopic sphincterotomy if papillary stenosis is present, but antibiotics aimed at eradicating the underlying infection seem to be only rarely helpful.

Compared to ultrasonography, CT is slightly more sensitive but no more specific in detecting hepatic abnormalities. Thus a CT scan may show a lesion if the ultrasound is normal, but is unlikely to better define an abnormality already detected by ultrasound. On the other hand, CT is more accurate than ultrasonography in visualizing the retroperitoneum, the area of the abdomen where lymphoma especially tends to develop.

Diagnostic paracentesis is valuable in the setting of ascites without obvious cause.

Liver Biopsy in Diffuse Liver Disease

Several series have shown that liver biopsies show abnormalities in the vast majority of HIV patients with elevated liver enzymes and no mass lesions. However, most often biopsy demonstrates a condition that (1) is nonspecific and does not warrant treatment (e.g., steatosis, portal inflammation, congestion, granulomas without a pathogen), (2) is diagnosable by safer tests (blood tests for MAC), or (3) requires therapy only in unusual circumstances (Kaposi's sarcoma). Hepatic biopsies are most useful to determine the severity of chronic viral hepatitis, and in the setting of elevated liver enzymes with fever and normal chest x-ray, stool examination, blood culture, and bone marrow biopsy (searching for CMV hepatitis). If a biopsy is done, samples should be sent not only for routine histologic examination, but also for AFB stain, fungal stains, Warthin-Starry stain (for bacillary angiomatosis), immunohistochemistry, in situ hybridization, and mycobacterial, viral, and fungal cultures.

INDICATIONS FOR ADMISSION

Rapidly progressing liver disease, especially when associated with encephalopathy and/or an elevated prothrombin time/partial thromboplastin time is best managed in hospital. In other situations, investigations, including liver biopsy, can be arranged on an outpatient basis.

ESOPHAGEAL DISEASE
Etiology

In HIV infection, there is a greater than 90 percent likelihood of esophageal infection or neoplasia when the patient complains of odynophagia (pain while swallowing), dysphagia (difficulty in swallowing), or substernal chest pain. The commonest condition is *Candida* infection of the esophagus, but esophageal ulceration from CMV and herpes is also frequent. Idiopathic esophageal ulceration, possibly caused by HIV itself, is being increasingly recognized. Less common entities are lymphoma, Kaposi's sarcoma, MAC, and drug-induced lesions. Peptic esophagitis also occurs, but is uncommon when the CD4 count is <100 since gastric acid secretion is usually diminished in these patients.

Investigations

Both general clinical experience and the literature (including a prospective trial) indicate that endoscopy is significantly more sensitive and accurate than barium contrast radiography, even in expert hands. There is less of a consensus about whether all patients with esophageal symptoms should undergo immediate diagnostic endoscopy, or whether they should first be given an empiric trial of treatment for *Candida* esophagitis. A decision analysis shows that the most cost-effective strategy is empiric therapy with fluconazole 200 mg daily for presumed *Candida,* followed by endoscopy if there is no response in 2 weeks. However, U.S. data were used in this report, and when

Canadian endoscopy and drug costs are considered, a definite diagnosis with initial flexible esophagogastroduodenoscopy turns out to be efficient. Oropharyngeal candidiasis (thrush) is associated with a higher prevalence of esophageal *Candida*. Thus in this population, a 2-week *trial* of empiric antifungal therapy makes sense, but in all other circumstances endoscopy is advisable since an accurate diagnosis cannot be made from symptoms alone. Mucosal biopsy of all visible lesions is recommended; biopsies should ideally be sent to for routine histology, in situ hybridization, and virology. CMV is sometimes difficult to diagnose, since isolation of the virus from a mucosal biopsy can be due to just contamination from blood or saliva. Hence CMV effect detected histologically is the key diagnostic feature. If endoscopy shows no abnormalities, biopsies are not necessary (since they always turn out to be normal), and esophageal motility studies should be considered.

Treatment

Hospital admission is necessary only if the esophageal symptoms are so that severe dehydration and/or malnutrition have developed.

Treatment options for esophageal candidiasis include topical agents such as clotrimazole, miconazole, and nystatin. However, oral ketoconazole 200 to 400 mg/day, itraconazole 100 mg/day, or fluconazole 100 to 200 mg/day are more commonly used. Ketoconazole is relatively inexpensive, but side effects have been reported, including liver disease, inhibition of adrenal/testicular steroidogenesis, and interaction with rifampin. Gastric acid is necessary for optimal ketoconazole absorption, and therefore hydrochloric acid should be concomitantly administered to patients with a low CD4 count (since hypochlorhydria is common in AIDS). A randomized trial has found fluconazole 100 mg/day more effective than ketoconazole 200 mg/day in resolving symptoms and eradicating *Candida* from the esophagus.

Fungal esophageal infections refractory to oral medications can be due to non-*Candida* species, such as *Torulopsis glabrata,* to poor drug compliance/drug bioavailability, or to *Candida albicans* resistant to imidazole drugs (which include ketoconazole, fluconazole, and itraconazole). Fluconazole-resistant infections require IV amphotericin.

In HIV, fungal esophageal infections almost never become systemic, unlike in other immunocompromised hosts. Accordingly, aggressive therapy is necessary only if the symptoms are severe.

Follow-up studies have shown that *Candida* esophagitis almost invariably recurs, usually within 12 weeks of a successful treatment response. Maintenance treatment can prevent such recurrences, but is not recommended since this risks the development of resistant strains. Furthermore, the cost:benefit ratio of suppressive therapy is very high in view of the rarity of *Candida* spread outside the esophagus. One reasonable approach is to simply provide to the patient a supply of the antifungal drug that eradicated the first *Candida* infection, and ask the patient to take the drug whenever esophageal symptoms develop.

CMV and herpes esophagitis are treated with antiviral drugs, as described elsewhere in this book. A satisfactory response can be expected from ganciclovir or foscarnet, although the recurrence rate has been reported to be 40 percent within 18 months. Similarly, acyclovir almost always heals herpetic esophageal ulcers. Kaposi's sarcoma is often asymptomatic, in which case treatment is not advised; otherwise management is the same as for such lesions appearing in other organs. Laser coagulation has also been described as effective.

Idiopathic ulceration usually requires prednisone at a starting dose of 40 mg/day. Other reported therapies include thalidomide, endoscopic injection of the ulcers with corticosteroids, and discontinuing zidovudine and didanosine. A relapse rate of almost 25 percent has been reported after successful therapy, with even higher rates if corticosteroids are given for less than 1 month.

Suggested Readings

ABDOMINAL PAIN

Benhamou Y, Housset C, Dumont JL, et al. AIDS-related cholangiopathy: critical analysis of a prospective series of 26 patients. Dig Dis Sci 1993;38:1113–8.

Parente F, Cerrnuschi M, Antinori S, et al. Severe abdominal pain in patients with AIDS: frequency, clinical aspects, causes, and outcomes. Scad J Gastroentrol 1994;29:511–5.

Thuluvath PJ, Connolly GM, Forbes A, Gazzard BG. Abdominal pain in HIV infection. Q J Med 1991;78:275–85.

DIARRHEA

Dieterich DT, Kotler DP, Busch DF, et al. Ganciclovir treatment of cytomegalovirus colitis in AIDS: a randomized double-blind, placebo-controlled multicenter study. J Infect Dis 1993;167:278–82.

Kotler DP. Gastrointestinal manifestations of human immunodeficiency virus infection. Adv Intern Med 1995;40:197–242.

Petri WA, Clark CG, Diamond LS. Host–parasite relationships in amebiasis: conference report. J Infect Dis 1994;169:483–4.

Mayer HB, Wanke CA. Diagnostic strategies in HIV-infected patients with diarrhea. AIDS 1994;8:16399–48.

Rabeneck L. Diagnostic work-up strategies for patients with HIV-related chronic diarrhea. J Clin Gastroenterol 1993;16: 245–50.

Simon D, Brandt LJ. Diarrhea in patients with the acquired immune deficiency syndrome. Gastroenterology 1993;105:1238–42.

Simon DM, Cello JP, Valenzuela J, et al. Multicenter trial of octreotide in patients with refractory acquired immunodeficiency syndrome-associated diarrhea. Gastroenterology 1995; 108:1753–60.

ELEVATED LIVER ENZYMES

Bonacini M. Hepatobiliary complications in patients with human immunodeficiency virus infection. Am J Med 1992; 92: 404–11.

Cello JP. Human immunodeficiency virus-associated biliary tract disease. Semin Liver Dis 1992;12:213–8.

Scharschmidt BF, Held MJ, Hollander HH, et al. Hepatitis B in patients with HIV infection: relationship to AIDS and patient survival. Ann Intern Med 1992; 117:837–8.

Schneiderman DJ, Arenson DM, Cello JP, et al. Hepatic disease in patients with acquired immune deficiency syndrome (AIDS). Hepatology 1987; 7:925–30.

ESOPHAGEAL DISEASE

Laine L. The natural history of esophageal Candidiasis after successful treatment in patients with AIDS. Gastroenterology 1994; 107:744–6.

Laine L, Bonacini M. Esophageal disease in human immunodeficiency syndrome. Arch Intern Med 1994; 154:1577–82.

Laine L, Dretler RH, Conteas CN, et al. Fluconazole compared with ketoconazole for the treatment of Candida esophagitis in AIDS. Ann Intern Med 1992; 117: 655–60.

Wilcox CM, Schwartz DA. Comparison of two corticosteroid regimens for the treatment of HIV-associated idiopathic esophageal ulcer. Am J Gastroenterol 1994; 89: 2163–7.

Wilcox CM, Schwartz DA, Clark WS. Esophageal ulceration in human immunodeficiency virus infection. Ann Intern Med 1995; 123: 143–9.

Wilcox CM, Straub RF, Schwartz DA. Cytomegalovirus esophagitis in AIDS: A prospective evaluation of clinical response to ganciclovir therapy, relapse rate, and long term outcome. Am J Med 1995; 98:169–76.

CENTRAL NERVOUS SYSTEM MANIFESTATIONS

NEUROLOGICAL PRESENTATIONS

Krystyna Ostrowska, M.D., F.R.C.P.C.

Clinical Presentation

Because of its neurotropic properties, the human immunodeficiency virus invades the central nervous system (CNS) early in the course of infection. In 70 percent of cases, the initial CNS invasion is asymptomatic. In the remaining 30 percent, acute aseptic meningitis may develop within days to weeks after seroconversion, presenting acutely or subacutely as focal or diffuse encephalitis. Meningitis with headache, nuchal rigidity, and ataxia or myelopathy is typical. Palsies of cranial nerves V, VII, and VIII may be present. The cerebrospinal fluid (CSF) shows mild lymphocytic or mononuclear pleocytosis, normal or slightly lower glucose, and elevated protein. Aseptic meningitis can also occur later in the asymptomatic phase at CD_4 counts of between 200 and 500. Most patients recover spontaneously within weeks, but some may be left with permanent cognitive deficits.

During the asymptomatic period between seroconversion and the development of AIDS, CSF abnormalities persist. Cell count, protein, and immunoglobulins are usually slightly elevated. Such abnormalities most likely represent HIV invasion of the CSF unless an alternative etiology is found (such as a positive serologic test for syphilis). Late CNS complications do not occur until CD_4 counts drop to <200.

At this stage, 30 to 40 percent of patients have neurologic complications as the chief presenting feature of AIDS. At autopsy, 75 percent of all AIDS patients show some neurologic involvement.

Clinical manifestations vary from meningitis and focal CNS lesions to diffuse brain disease with or without changes in the level of consciousness. Diagnostic tests may include CT/magnetic resonance imaging, lumbar puncture with culture, brain biopsy, and neuropsychiatric testing. Figures 8–1 to 8–4 present the evaluation and management of several CNS manifestations of CNS disease in HIV/AIDS. The text continues following the algorithms on page 106.

CHANGE IN MENTAL STATUS

Alterness

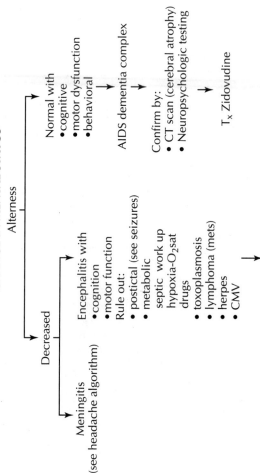

Decreased

Meningitis
(see headache algorithm)

Encephalitis with
• cognition
• motor function

Rule out:
• postictal (see seizures)
• metabolic
  septic work up
  hypoxia-O_2sat
  drugs
• toxoplasmosis
• lymphoma (mets)
• herpes
• CMV

Normal with
• cognitive
• motor dysfunction
• behavioral

AIDS dementia complex

Confirm by:
• CT scan (cerebral atrophy)
• Neuropsychologic testing

T_x Zidovudine

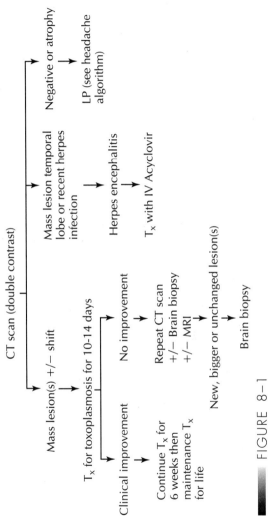

FIGURE 8–1
Evaluation and Management of Changes in Mental Status

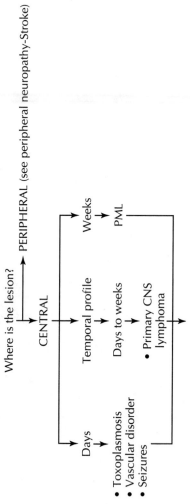

FOCAL NEUROLOGICAL DEFICIT

Where is the lesion?

PERIPHERAL (see peripheral neuropathy-Stroke)

CENTRAL

Temporal profile

Days →
- Toxoplasmosis
- Vascular disorder
- Seizures

Days to weeks →
- Primary CNS lymphoma

Weeks → PML

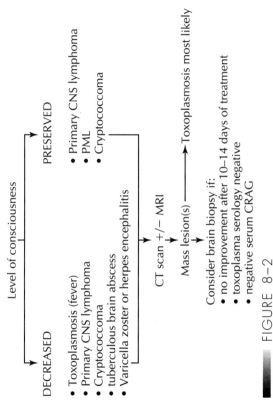

FIGURE 8–2
Evaluation and Management of Focal Neurologic Deficit

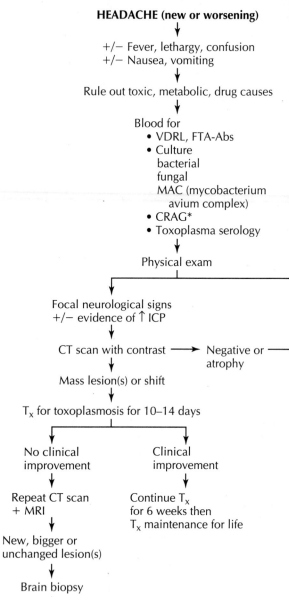

HEADACHE (new or worsening)

+/− Fever, lethargy, confusion
+/− Nausea, vomiting

Rule out toxic, metabolic, drug causes

Blood for
- VDRL, FTA-Abs
- Culture
  bacterial
  fungal
  MAC (mycobacterium
  avium complex)
- CRAG*
- Toxoplasma serology

Physical exam

Focal neurological signs
+/− evidence of ↑ ICP

CT scan with contrast ⟶ Negative or atrophy

Mass lesion(s) or shift

T_x for toxoplasmosis for 10–14 days

No clinical improvement   Clinical improvement

Repeat CT scan + MRI   Continue T_x for 6 weeks then T_x maintenance for life

New, bigger or unchanged lesion(s)

Brain biopsy

* Cryptococcal antigen test

FIGURE 8–3

Evaluation and Management of New or Worsening Headache

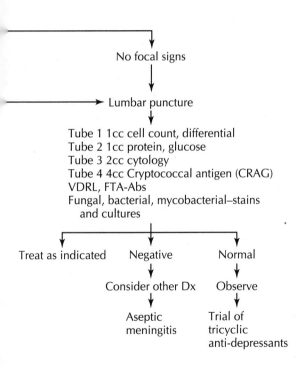

No focal signs

Lumbar puncture

Tube 1 1cc cell count, differential
Tube 2 1cc protein, glucose
Tube 3 2cc cytology
Tube 4 4cc Cryptococcal antigen (CRAG)
VDRL, FTA-Abs
Fungal, bacterial, mycobacterial–stains
  and cultures

Treat as indicated   Negative   Normal

Consider other Dx   Observe

Aseptic   Trial of
meningitis   tricyclic
  anti-depressants

SEIZURES

Control status epilepticus or generalized seizures, then investigate the cause

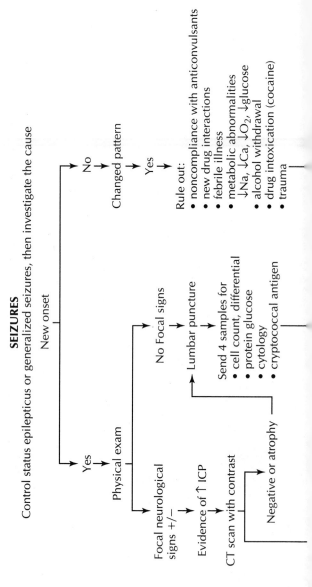

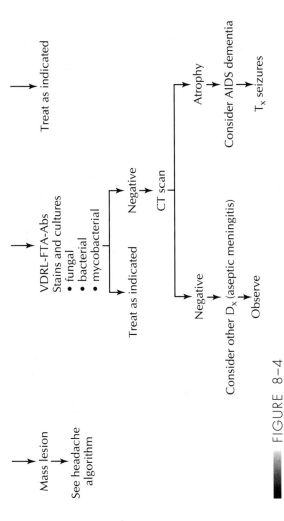

FIGURE 8-4
Evaluation and Management of Seizures

Differential Diagnosis

The differential diagnosis of the most common clinical presentations is listed below:

Meningitis

- Aseptic (HIV?)
- Cryptococcal
- Asymptomatic meningeal reaction
- Tuberculous
- Syphilitic
- *Histoplasmosis*
- *Coccidioidomycosis*
- Lymphomatous (metastatic)

Focal Lesions

- CNS toxoplasmosis
- Primary CNS lymphoma
- Progressive multifocal leukoencephalopathy
- Tuberculous brain abscess
- Cryptococcoma
- Varicella-zoster encephalitis
- Herpes encephalitis
- Gumma

Diffuse Brain Disease

- Encephalopathies with depressed level of consciousness
  —Metabolic
  —Toxoplasmosis
  —CMV
  —Herpes

- Dementias
  —AIDS dementia complex

NEUROMUSCULAR COMPLICATIONS
Ronald MacDonald, M.D., F.R.C.P.C.

Neuromuscular complications of HIV infection occur in 10 to 20 percent of HIV-infected patients and may herald its diagnosis. The most common causes include the following:

- Distal sensory motor neuropathy.
- Acute inflammatory polyneuropathy (Guillain-Barré syndrome).
- Chronic inflammatory polyneuropathy.
- Mononeuritis multiplex.
- Polyradiculopathy (CMV).
- Myopathy.

Distal Symmetrical Peripheral Neuropathy

This problem is signalled by burning pain and numbness of the soles of the feet. On physical examination, ankle jerks are absent. A moderate decrease of all sensory modalities with eventual loss of lower limb sensation is found. Motor involvement varies from mild to severe. The course varies and may involve remission, stabilization, or a relentlessly progressive advance.

Investigations include electromyography (EMG), which shows axonal neuropathy. The etiology is not yet certain, but may include direct HIV invasion or immunopathology or a secondary process due to toxic (e.g., didanosine [ddI], zalcitabine [ddC], staduvine [d4T]) and metabolic or nutritional factors. Therapy with steroids or plasmapheresis offers little help. Zidovudine (AZT) may improve symptoms in some cases. Treatment of neuropathic pain with amitryptyline or carbamazepine may offer symptomatic relief.

Acute and Chronic Demyelinating Neuropathy

This condition, often the presenting illness of HIV infection, is indistinguishable from idiopathic demyelinating neuropathy. On physical examination, the patient is areflexic, and has motor weakness, facial diplegia, and respiratory involvement. On lumbar puncture, the CSF protein is increased and a lymphocytic pleocytosis may be seen. The pathogenesis is unknown. Treatment with plasmapheresis is effective and prognosis is good.

Mononeuritis Multiplex

The neuropathy often starts abruptly, with multiple peripheral nerves and cranial nerves III, IV, V, and VII affected. Symptoms may resolve spontaneously or progress to a polyneuropathy. Pathogenesis is unknown but vasculitis may be implicated. Steroid therapy is of no use.

Progressive Polyradiculopathy

This condition is rare and is usually confined to L5 roots (cauda equina). The onset is subacute, with motor and sensory involvement, early sphincter involvement, and sacral sensory loss. The course is relentlessly progressive. Lumbar puncture should be performed. CSF examination will demonstrate pleocytosis, increased protein, and decreased glucose. CMV is the most likely cause. Treatment with ganciclovir is recommended, although is of questionable benefit.

HIV-Associated Myopathy

The presentation is most often subacute. Proximal weakness is noted, linked to increased creatine kinase. Occasionally myopathy is seen with prolonged zidovudine therapy. EMG shows a myopathic picture and muscle biopsy reveals fiber necrosis and inflammatory infiltrates. The pathogenesis is unknown, as HIV has not been isolated from muscle. The response to therapy with immunosuppression is variable, and 50 percent improve with steroid therapy.

Suggested Readings

Management of neurologic opportunistic disorders in human immunodeficiency virus infection. Semin Neurol 1992; 12 (No. 1), 28–33.

McArthur JC. Neurologic manifestations of AIDS. Medicine 1987; 66 (No. 6), 407–32.

Price RW, Worley JM. Management of neurologic complications of HIV-1 infection and AIDS. In Sande MA, Volberding PA (eds). The Medical Management of AIDS. 4th ed. Philadelphia: WB Saunders, 1995.

■■■ FEVER

Mary Fanning, M.D., P.h.D., F.R.C.P.C., F.A.C.P.

Fevers, or temperatures ≥38.0°C, are very common in HIV-infected patients and their causes vary according to the stage of disease. They arise from numerous conditions and often occur together with other symptoms that may help to elucidate the cause, such as shortness of breath in patients with PCP. However, many patients present just with fever and a careful work-up may reveal a treatable underlying reason. The most common causes are CMV disease and mycobacterial infections such as MAC or tuberculosis. Less frequent causes of fever include salmonellosis; histoplasmosis; unusual presentations of common focal infections such as PCP, toxoplasmosis, and cryptococcosis; non-Hodgkin's lymphomas; and complications of IV drug use or sexually transmitted diseases such as syphilis.

In some cases, however, a diagnosis of HIV-associated fever is made by exclusion, after completing all the appropriate investigations listed below. An unexplained fever of ≥38.5°C for more than 4 weeks, in association with other findings such as weight loss and night sweats, constitutes Centers for Disease Control and Prevention stage IVa HIV disease.

When fever is the first presenting symptom, a careful history and physical examination is necessary. The initial evaluation should try to identify a localizing source (e.g., PCP, IV catheter infection, bacterial pneumonia or sinus infection). The history should include information about IV drug use and sexual activity, since sepsis, bacterial endocarditis, or syphilis may produce fever. A careful history of medications taken is also essential. Fever may also signify early allergic reactions to drugs such as TMP-SMX (Septra), before a skin rash emerges.

Basic investigations include a CBC, blood and urine cultures, and a chest x-ray. The physical examination should be thorough, with special attention to the skin, mouth, chest, CNS, and reticuloendothelial system.

CD4 COUNT >200 OR 20 PERCENT

Basic investigations include a careful physical examination, CBC, chest x-ray, urinalysis, blood chemistries, serologic test for syphilis, and blood and urine cultures. Further investigation and management depend on the initial results.

CD4 COUNT <200 OR 20 PERCENT

In addition to the above work-up, blood is cultured for mycobacteria and fungi. Serum cryptococcal antigen should be measured if headache is present or if fever lasts more than 2 weeks with negative initial investigations. Blood and urine cultures for CMV are frequently positive in individuals without CMV disease because of viral shedding. Diagnosis of CMV requires an ophthalmologic examination for typical lesions or tissue biopsy with electron microscopic demonstration of inclusion bodies, positive fluorescent staining for CMV, or a positive tissue culture.

If the patient is clinically ill, hospitalization may be required for further investigations, including lumbar puncture, bone marrow aspirate, and biopsy for culture (bacterial, mycobacterial, and fungal) and pathology. CT scans of the brain may be needed to rule out toxoplasmosis, and a careful fundoscopic examination to detect CMV disease is essential.

PREVIOUS DIAGNOSIS OF AIDS

The likelihood of opportunistic infections due to MAC, toxoplasmosis, cryptococcosis, CMV, and lymphoma is greatly increased in AIDS patients and investigation to rule out these conditions should be pursued.

MAC	Blood cultures for mycobacteria
Toxoplasmosis	Serum antibody titer CNS CT scan
Cryptococcosis	Serum cryptococcal antigen Chest X-ray Lumbar puncture for India ink preparation Cryptococcal antigen and culture
CMV	Ophthalmologic examination Biopsy of esophagus or colon if gastrointestinal symptoms suggestive of CMV are present
Lymphoma	CNS and abdominal CT scans

NEUTROPENIA

A febrile patient with a neutrophil count of <500 requires prompt attention regardless of the cause of neutropenia. Such patients should be admitted and have three sets of blood cultures drawn. Broad-spectrum antibiotics (e.g., cefazolin and gentamicin/tobramycin) should be started.

Suggested Reading

Dulrack DT, Street AC. Fever of unknown origin re-examined and redefined. Curr Clin Topics Infect Dis 1991; 11: 35–51.

MUSCULOSKELETAL COMPLICATIONS

Dafna Gladman, M.D., F.R.C.P.C.

Recently recognized musculoskeletal complications of HIV infection include arthralgias (which present as joint pain without evidence of inflammation) and AIDS-associated arthritis (an inflammatory arthritis involving primarily large joints). Spondyloarthropathies, including Reiter syndrome, psoriatic spondyloarthropathy, and an undifferentiated spondyloarthropathy have also been described. Sjögren syndrome, consisting of dry eyes, dry mouth, and arthritis, has been diagnosed among patients with HIV infection, as well as other collagen diseases, including polymyositis and miscellaneous vasculitides. Many patients, particularly those treated with zidovudine (AZT), present with muscle weakness, which may be a side effect of the treatment. Fibromyalgia has recently been documented in as many as 30 percent of patients with HIV infection. In addition, septic arthritis and osteomyelitis may occur.

The evaluation and management of joint pain in the HIV-infected patient is presented in Figure 8-5. When a patient with HIV infection presents with joint pain, the first step is to assess whether there is active inflammation, and whether it is localized to the joint. Joint inflammation is usually associated with stiffness and swelling, and occasionally with redness. There is often associated morning stiffness. When joint inflammation is noted, causative infection must be excluded. Patients with HIV, particularly those on therapy, may be predisposed to infection, and septic arthritis is common among AIDS patients. If the joint is swollen, it must be aspirated and the synovial fluid removed and cultured. Sources of infection should be sought, such as an open wound, or infection at other sites. Septic arthritis requires prompt treatment with IV antibiotics in order to avoid joint destruction and the development of osteomyelitis. The latter should be suspected when there is bone pain and/or swelling beyond the joint. Patients suspected of septic arthritis or osteomyelitis should be admitted to hospital for treatment. Osteomyelitis may be confirmed by a technetium bone scan followed by a gallium scan. In osteomyelitis, the gallium scan is "hotter" than the technetium scan. A biopsy may be necessary to confirm the diagnosis, and to identify the infecting organism, in order to provide more appropriate

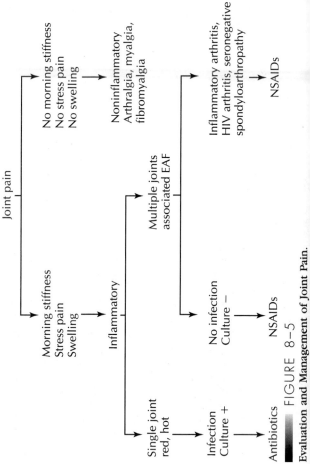

FIGURE 8–5

Evaluation and Management of Joint Pain.

antimicrobial therapy. While the most common causative agents remain staphylococci and streptococci, unusual organisms may be seen in this particular population.

▪▪▪▪ NUTRITION

Maggie Jane Marchand, B.Sc.

Nutrition plays a vital role in immune system function. Protein-calorie malnutrition may decrease both the total number and function of the T-lymphocytes, is known to reduce cellular immunity, and results in atrophy of the vital organs involved in immune system function, including the thymus. Nutrient deficiencies, excesses, and imbalances also have a detrimental influence on various components of the immune system (Table 8–9). Therefore, in immune-compromised individuals, nutrition plays a key part of the treatment plan.

Progressive weight loss and debilitation commonly accompany HIV infection. The course of AIDS is often complicated by profound weight loss, cachexia, and multiple nutrient deficiencies—particularly protein-calorie malnutrition. As the disease progresses, the nutritional status of people with HIV is undermined by nutrient malabsorption, diarrhea, anorexia, oral/esophageal problems including candidiasis, nausea, vomiting, and infection. The multifactorial nature of AIDS produces a different combination of

TABLE 8–9

Micronutrients Associated with Immune System Defects or Increased Infection Susceptibility

Vitamin A
Vitamin B$_6$
Vitamin B$_{12}$
Vitamin C
Vitamin E
Thiamin
Riboflavin
Zinc
Copper
Iron
Selenium
Essential fatty acids

symptoms in each individual. Food intake may be restricted by a decreased appetite, fatigue which may limit both shopping and meal preparation abilities, alterations in taste perception, or gastrointestinal intolerances secondary to the side effects of medications for HIV disease. Hence, malnutrition is now being proposed as a potential cofactor in the progression of HIV disease.

Despite the use of antiretroviral medications, prophylaxis and therapy against many of the major opportunistic infections, for example, PCP, MAC, the incidence of weight loss and wasting is increasing. HIV wasting syndrome was included by the Centers for Disease Control and Prevention in 1987 as an AIDS-defining illness. It is defined as an involuntary weight loss of >10 percent baseline body weight plus either chronic diarrhea (at least two loose bowel movements per day for >30 days) or chronic weakness and documented fever (≥30 days, intermittent or constant) in the absence of a concurrent illness or condition other than HIV infection that would explain the findings.

As with any chronic disease, the severe malnutrition that frequently accompanies AIDS can negatively influence survival rates/times. In addition, the quality of life for people with HIV/AIDS can be seriously compromised if their main illness is further affected by nutritional complications. (Fig. 8–6)

Nutritional counselling and intervention should begin as soon as an individual is diagnosed as HIV positive, so that

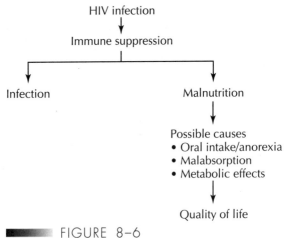

FIGURE 8-6
Proposed Concept of Nutrition in HIV/AIDS.

the potential dangers of malnutrition may be addressed early in the infection. The key goals of nutritional intervention are to optimize nutritional status and provide support to optimize immune system function.

GOALS OF NUTRITIONAL INTERVENTION IN HIV-POSITIVE PATIENTS

HIV-Positive Asymptomatic Patients

1. Achieve and maintain optimal nutritional status.
2. Encourage healthy eating habits, weight maintenance, and lean muscle mass development/maintenance.
3. Encourage patient involvement in active exercise programs—aerobic and resistance training.
4. Discuss the pros and cons of popular "fad diets" and "complementary/alternate therapies" to help patients make well-informed decisions.
5. Review vitamin/mineral supplementation programs.
6. Review food safety guidelines to decrease the risk of food-borne illness or opportunistic infections.

AIDS Patients

Goals for this group may include the goals outlined previously, plus the following:

1. Aim to prevent weight loss and maintain lean muscle mass.
2. Aim to provide adequate levels of all nutrients—protein, calories, fluids, vitamins, minerals.
3. Minimize symptoms of malabsorption and gastrointestinal conditions that may compromise nutritional intake/status.
4. Aim to support nutritional status in order for the patient to maximize quality of life.

NUTRITIONAL STATUS ASSESSMENT IN HIV/AIDS PATIENTS

The foundation of nutritional support is based on the nutritional status assessment. Nutritional assessment components are as follows:

- Diet history.
- Social, behavioral, and economic factors.
- Medical history/opportunistic infections and nutritional implications.
- Drug–nutrient interactions/side effects of medications (Table 8–10).
- Physical and anthropometric indices.
- Weight history, including body mass index.
- Laboratory values–biochemical data.

When a patient is admitted to hospital the following should be ordered:

- High-protein, high-calorie diet: dietitian to consult.
- Weight: initially and then every Monday and Thursday.
- Height.
- Serum albumin and TIBC: initially and then every week to assess protein status and nutritional repletion/depletion.
- Serum cholesterol and triglycerides: important if patient on antiviral therapy (didanosine [ddI]/zalcitabine [ddC] to assess the risk of increased lipid level (triglyceride)-associated pancreatitis.
- Hemoglobin/hematocrit: to assess anemia.

NUTRITION MANAGEMENT: CURRENT RECOMMENDATIONS

The following nutrient recommendations are suggested as guidelines and *must* be individualized for each patient.

Calories

May be estimated using the Harris–Benedict equation, with allowances for activity and stress.
Males:

$$66.5 + 13.8 \text{ (weight in kg)} + 5.0 \text{ (height in cm)} - 6.8 \text{ (age)}$$

Females:

$$665.1 + 9.6 \text{ (weight in kg)} + 1.8 \text{ (height in cm)} - 4.7 \text{ (age)}$$

Quick estimate: 35 to 45 Kcal/Kg usual body weight (UBWt).

TABLE 8-10 ▬▬▬▬▬▬▬▬▬▬▬

Nutritional Concerns/Implications of Selected Drugs Used to Treat HIV Illness

DRUG	POTENTIAL FOOD/NUTRIENT CONCERNS
Acyclovir	Diarrhea, nausea, vomiting, anorexia, metallic taste, headache, hypotension
Amphotericin B	Metallic taste, weight loss, nausea, vomiting, diarrhea, anorexia, possible decreased serum potassium, magnesium Metallic taste
Zidovudine (AZT, Retrovir)	Possible nausea, anorexia, constipation Vomiting, diarrhea, taste alterations Need to monitor for anemia: possible B_{12} folate deficiency Muscle atrophy: avoid with fatty meals
Didanosine (ddI, Videx)	May result in elevated triglycerides, possible pancreatitis No alcohol Requires a basic/alkaline media for absorption
Dapsone (Avlosulfon)	Anorexia, sore throat, anemia, abdominal pain
Foscarnet	Nausea, anorexia, increased thirst Potential hypocalcemia (rare)
Ganciclovir	Possible nausea, anorexia, anemia Oral form should be taken with food
Isoniazid (INH)	Possible hyperglycemia, dry mouth, nausea, vomiting, anorexia Folate antagonist: evaluate dietary folate B_6 antagonist: give 25 mg pyridoxine daily Empty stomach may increase absorption
Fluconazole	Nausea, vomiting, abdominal pain Possible increase in transaminases
Ketoconazole	Possible nausea, vomiting, abdominal pain; watch for hyponatremia To enhance absorption take with acidic beverage (e.g., cola, orange juice) Do not administer with antacids

(Continued)

TABLE 8–10

Nutritional Concerns/Implications of Selected Drugs Used to Treat HIV Illness (Continued)

DRUG	POTENTIAL FOOD/NUTRIENT CONCERNS
Megestrol acetate (Megace)	Increased appetite, weight gain, constipation, mild edema
Nystatin	Diarrhea, nausea, vomiting Take on empty stomach: avoid eating for ½ hour after treatment to increase mucosal contact time
IV pentamidine	Possible hypoglycemia even after therapy discontinues Possible hyperglycemia May cause nausea, vomiting, diarrhea, sore throat, anorexia, metallic taste, dry mouth Hyperkalemia on IV drug Hypocalcemia Folate deficiency
Pyrimethamine	Requires folinic acid supplement
Rizampin	Nausea, vomiting, anorexia Empty stomach may increase absorption
Sulfadiazine	Possible GI upset, nausea, vomiting, diarrhea Take with water
Trimethoprim-sulfamethoxizole (TMP-SM, Bactim, Septra)	Possible anorexia, nausea, diarrhea, stomatitis May decrease folate absorption, check blood folate levels Take with water to maintain adequate hydration
Ciprofloxacin	Minimize caffeine intake Milk, dairy products, nutritional supplements and mineral supplements may decrease absorption
Rifabutin	Possible GI side effects Nausea, vomiting
Humatin	GI upset
Atovaquone (Mepron)	GI upset, diarrhea Take with fatty foods to increase absorption

Protein

Quick estimate: 1.2 to 1.5 g/Kg UBWt; must consider liver and renal function (to allow for repletion with no acute infection).

Fiber

A higher-fiber diet is required in patients with constipation related to pain medication. The type of fiber (soluble or insoluble) may be adjusted in cases of diarrhea.

Micronutrients

There are currently no documented scientific investigations that have clearly defined guidelines on the use of vitamins and minerals in HIV infection.

As a general guideline, it is suggested that multivitamin/mineral supplements not exceed 200 percent of the recommended nutrient intake. Use of additional supplements should be discussed/reviewed with the patient; in large doses micronutrients may have toxic effects, as indicated below:

- Vitamin C: kidney stones, rebound scurvy, gastrointestinal distress.
- Vitamin B_6: neurotoxicity.
- Vitamin A: gastrointestinal distress, hepatic dysfunction.
- Copper: gastrointestinal distress.
- Zinc: copper deficiency, gastrointestinal and cardiac effects.

Studies by Abrams et al.[1] and Tang et al.[2] suggest a link between a reduction in the rate of HIV progression and nutrient intake. Abrams et al. examined the relationship between dietary intakes and the progression to AIDS. In a 6-year prospective study involving 296 subjects, the daily use of a multivitamin was associated with a 31 percent decrease in the advancement to an AIDS-defining illness. The intake of iron, zinc, folate, thiamin, niacin, riboflavin, ascorbic acid, and vitamins A and E were analyzed. Iron, vitamin E, and riboflavin intake appear to play a statistically protective role.

In the second study by Tang et al., participants were monitored for their usual and daily dietary supplement intake every 6 months. Over the median 6.8-year follow-up period, in the 281 subjects, highest intakes of vitamin C, thiamin, and niacin were associated with a significantly decreased progression rate to AIDS.

At this time there is no conclusive evidence to confirm that megadosing of vitamins or minerals will alter the course of HIV infection/progression.

The area of optimal vitamin/mineral supplementation will likely continue to provide much debate and controversy for health care practitioners and patients. Further investigations are essential to help address the many unanswered questions.

MANAGEMENT OF SYMPTONS AND CONDITIONS

Anorexia/Weight Loss

- Individualized meal plans: change to six small meals, including favorite foods to encourage intake.
- High-protein, high-calorie diet: may include commercial calorically dense supplements (e.g., Boost, Ensure, Resource).
- Snacking.
- Limited use of low-calorie foods with limited nutritive value (e.g., coffee, tea).
- Monitoring of body weight changes and serum protein levels.
- Appetite stimulants (e.g., megetrol acetate [Megace], dronabinol [Marinol], see below).
- Tube feeding when energy and protein requirements cannot be provided by oral intake (12-hour nocturnal feeds recommended to maximize oral intake during the day).

Disorders of the Oral/Esophageal Cavity

- Modification of diet consistency, texture, and temperature to maximize intake. Soft, nonirritating foods (e.g., pasta dishes, eggs, ground beef).
- Sauces/gravy to moisten meals.
- Foods at cool temperature for patients with oral lesions.
- Avoidance of spicy, acidic, or abrasive foods.
- Nutrient-dense supplements.
- Good oral hygiene, especially if oral candidiasis is an issue.
- Blenderized/pureed meals, if patient has severe oral pain.

- Use of topical anesthetics to relieve discomfort.
- With swallowing difficulties, use of thickened liquids to decrease the risk of aspiration of thin beverages.
- If oral intake is extremely poor, enteral tube feedings to meet nutritional requirements.
- Total parenteral nutrition for severe esophageal ulceration.

Changes in Taste Perceptions

- Plastic utensils if food tastes metallic.
- Change in the temperature of meals served: (e.g., cold foods).
- Spices and flavorings.
- Good oral hygiene.

Nausea and Vomiting

- Avoidance of greasy, high-fat and spicy foods.
- Crackers, dry cereal, or toast in the morning.
- Clear liquids between meals.
- Small, frequent meals.
- Elimination of foods with strong aromas.
- Antiemetic drugs.
- Alteration of dosage and timing of drugs that may cause nausea.
- With vomiting, replacement of fluids and electrolytes with juices, soups, or sports drinks.
- When oral intake remains suboptimal for 7 days, short-term parenteral nutrition.

Infection and Sepsis

- "Energy-dense" oral supplements and/or initiation of tube feeding to meet increased needs.
- Adjustment of estimates of energy need for the febrile individual (7 percent increase in basal energy expenditure for every degree centigrade of body temperature over normal).

Neurologic Disease

- May result in reduced appetite, impaired ability to self-feed, and altered metabolic activity.

- Involvement of family/care givers and medical staff in the decision to provide nonvolitional support in people with severe dementia and a poor prognosis.

Diarrhea

- Identification of the cause of the diarrhea, if possible, so that appropriate medical treatments can be initiated.
- Replacement fluids/electrolytes.
- Decrease in sources of "roughage" (insoluble fibers), such as whole grain/bran products, nuts, raw fruit, and vegetables.
- Increase in sources of "pectin", (soluble fibers) such as applesauce, bananas, oatmeal, barley, dry toast/crackers, mashed potatoes, and rice.
- Avoidance of irritants and substances that decrease gastrointestinal transit time (e.g., alcohol, coffee, tea, chocolate, carbonated beverages).
- Avoidance/limitation of foods that may cause gas (beans, broccoli, cabbage, onions, cauliflower, peppers, cucumber, beer).
- Avoidance of extremes in temperature: foods/beverages served at room temperature.
- If steatorrhea is a problem, reduction of fats (butter, fried foods, pastries, sauces, salad dressings).
- Modification of lactose intake if milk/dairy products are a problem: lactose-reduced milk, small amounts of hard, aged cheese, and yogurt may be served to maintain some dairy intake based on patient tolerance.
- Antidiarrheal medication.
- Individualized nutritional care and careful monitoring because clinical manifestations vary among patients and in the same patient over time.
- For most patients with mild to moderate diarrhea or malabsorption the best diet is low in fat, lactose, and caffeine.
- Consultation with a dietitian: an elemental diet may be advised to help decrease severity of diarrhea.
- In cases of *Cryptosporidium* infection with total small-bowel disease, a course of parenteral nutrition to provide bowel rest and nutritional therapy secondary to severe malabsorption.

NUTRITIONAL SUPPORT OPTIONS

Appetite Stimulants

The use of various treatment modalities to help maintain nutritional status/weight is increasing as the negative implications of malnutrition on immune status and quality of life issues are further recognized.

The use of appetite stimulants is increasing as a standard of care in these patients. Megestrol acetate (Megace) and dronabinol (Marinol) are the two most common options.

Megesterol Acetate

Megesterol acetate (Megace), a synthetic orally active progestional agent, has been shown to stimulate appetite and promote weight gain. Patients have also reported an improved sense of well being/quality of life.

A variety of doses have been investigated: 100, 400, and 800 mg/day. Based on study results, 400 mg/day appears to be effective in promoting weight gain and has a lower incidence of potential dose-related side effects. These side effects may include edema, elevated blood glucose levels, and impotence.

Dronabinol (Marinol)

Dronabinol (Marinol) is an orally administered synthetic form of delta-9-tetrahydrocannabinol (THC). It has been used for anorexia and weight loss in patients with AIDS. The standard dose is 2.5 mg BID. A cannabinoid dose-related "high" (easy laughing, elation, and heightened awareness) has been reported in patients receiving dronabinol.

Patients on medications with CNS side effects, a history of cardiac disorders, substance abuse, or psychiatric conditions should be carefully evaluated before treatment is initiated and closely monitored while on this treatment.

Future Directions

New therapies, such as testerone replacement (based on the hormone's anabolic activity), anabolic steroids, including nandrolone decanoate (Deca-Durabolin), and thalidomide (may inhibit tumor necrosis factor, which may contribute to the anorexia), will likely receive further investigation in the near future.

Specialized Nutrition Support Options

The common standard of care for nutritional support in patients with HIV/AIDS is often structured on the following:

1. Nutritional assessment and counselling.

2. High-protein, calorically dense/fortified oral diet.

3. Step 2 plus use of liquid oral nutritional supplements.

4. Possible use of appetite stimulants, cytokine inhibitors, testosterone replacement therapy, or anabolic steroids (e.g., nandrolone decanoate) to promote weight gain.

For patients who have failed to respond or maintain their nutritional status on the approach outlined above, more active aggressive nutrition intervention may be indicated. Enteral and parenteral nutrition support are available options.

Enteral Nutrition

Enteral nutritional support refers to providing the body nutrients via the gastrointestinal tract. This may include short-term feeding via special tubes such as nasogastric or nasojejunal tubes. A surgically placed gastrostomy or jejunostomy is more appropriate for longer-term nutritional support. The use of the gastrointestinal tract for feeding is generally the preferred route. The continued use of the gastrointestinal tract supports its physiologic basis in helping to preserve gut function and maintain gastrointestinal mucosal integrity.

INDICATIONS FOR USE

1. Malnutrition with severe weight loss.

2. Inadequate oral intake to meet nutritional needs.

3. Esophageal or upper intestinal disease limiting oral intake (e.g., dysphagia, lymphoma, esophagitis).

CONTRAINDICATIONS

1. A nonfunctional gastrointestinal tract.

2. Complete or functional obstruction.

3. Intractable diarrhea.

FORMULA SELECTION

Based on gastrointestinal symptoms and degree of malabsorption:

1. Normal gastrointestinal function: intact/polymeric formula.

2. Bowel disease or malabsorption: elemental or peptide-based formula.

Once enteral feedings are initiated, patients should be monitored for tolerance, biochemical indices, fluid balance, and changes in nutritional status.

EFFICACY OF ENTERAL SUPPORT

At present there are limited studies dealing with the efficacy of enteral nutrition in HIV patients. In one study, Kotler[3] found improved nutritional status in eight severely ill, hospitalized HIV-positive patients fed via the enteral nutrition route. More research is required in this area to further define its role.

Parenteral Nutrition

Parenteral nutritional support refers to the intravenous provision of nutrients either via central (e.g., subclavian or peripheral veins).

INDICATIONS FOR USE

1. Severe diarrhea.
2. Intractable vomiting.
3. Severe gastrointestinal disease (e.g., intestinal obstruction, pancreatic inflammation/infection).

CONTRAINDICATIONS

A functional gastrointestinal tract that is capable of absorbing an adequate level of nutrients via an oral or enteral route.

Peripheral parenteral nutrition is appropriate for short-term use, usually less than 7 days. For long-term parenteral support a central access line is indicated. Protein, energy, fluids, and micronutrients (vitamins and minerals) can all be provided via the solution prescribed.

Patients on parenteral nutrition require close monitoring to ensure patient safety. Potential complications include problems associated with line placements (e.g., pneumothorax), biochemical abnormalities, and line infections.

The efficacy of parenteral nutrition support remains controversial and not clearly defined. Kotler[4] noted improvements and nutritional repletion in patients with malabsorption or eating disorders, but continued depletion in patients with systemic infections. Individual case histories in the literature have reported dramatic improvements in quality of life indices in selected individuals.

The decision to initiate more aggressive nutritional support therapies requires a multidisciplinary team approach and should actively involve patients/care givers, whose wishes should be respected. The efficacy of nutrition support and the development of support strategies is an area that should be of primary consideration among researchers.

References

1. Abrams B, et al. A prospective study of dietary intake and acquired immune deficiency syndrome in HIV-sero positive homosexual men. J AIDS 1993; 6: 949–58.
2. Tang AM, et al. Dietary micronutrient intake and risk of progression to acquired immunodeficiency syndrome (AIDS) in human immunodeficiency virus type 1 (HIV-1)-infected homosexual men. Am J Epidemiol 1993; 138: 937–51.
3. Kotler DP, et al. Enteral alimentation and repletion of body cell mass in malnourished patients with acquired immunodeficiency syndrome. Am J Clin Nutr 1991; 53: 149–54.
4. Kotler DP, et al. Total effect of home parenteral nutrition on body composition in patients with acquired immunodeficiency syndrome. Parenter Enter Nutr 1990; 14: 454–58.

Suggested Readings

Beal J. AIDS associated anorexia. J Phys Assoc AIDS Care 1995; 2 (No. 1): 19–23.
Coodley GO. The HIV wasting syndrome. A review. J AIDS 1994; 7: 681–94.
Galvin T. Micronutrients in human immunodeficiency virus disease. Top Clin Nutr 7: 3, 63–73.
Kotler DP (ed). Gastrointestinal and Nutritional Manifestations of the Acquired Immunodeficiency Syndrome. New York: Raven Press, 1991.
Murphy S. Healthy Eating makes a Difference. A Food Resource Book for People Living with HIV. Health and Welfare Canada, 1993.
Task Force on Nutrition Support in AIDS. Guidelines for nutrition support in AIDS. Nutrition 1989; 5:39–46.
Von Roenn JH, et al. Megestrol acetate in patients with AIDS-related cachexia. Ann Intern Med 1994; 121: 393–9.
Watson RR (ed). Nutrition and AIDS. Boca Raton, FL: CRC Press, 1994.

HEMATOLOGIC AND ONCOLOGIC MANIFESTATIONS

HEMATOLOGIC MANIFESTATIONS
Dale Dotten, M.D., F.R.C.P.C.

Viruses have long been associated with hematologic disorders. Recently, the human T-lymphocyte viruses (HTLV) have been associated with several hematologic disorders: HTLV-1 with T-cell chronic lymphocytic leukemia, HTLV-2 with hairy cell leukemia, and HTLV-3 (now termed HIV-1) with AIDS. The CD4 molecule is the major receptor for the HIV-1 virus, and thus CD4 cells including T-lymphocytes, monocytes, tissue macrophages, follicular dendritic cells, and megakaryocytes, are the predominant cells infected by the virus. The early CD34 progenitor cell does have a small number of CD4 surface molecules, but infection by the virus is likely of no clinical significance. However, infected stromal cells can transfect the later hematologic precursors. Although not conclusively proven, it is currently believed that the virus induces apoptosis, thus destroying the CD4 T-lymphocyte population. The interaction of the virus with the cell surface of CD34 cells may also induce apoptosis, and thus contributes to the decreased number of progenitor cells available. The hematologic abnormalities present reflect not only the effect of the virus per se, but also abnormalities in the modulation of hematopoiesis. Thus it is not surprising that intracellular modulator abnormalities, such as a decrease in erythropoeitin and granulocyte-macrophage colony stimulating factor (GM-CSF) and an increase in interleukin-6, have been documented.

Clinically, HIV infection can cause anemia, granulocytopenia, thrombocytopenia, or any combination thereof. It is important to recognize that, when confronted with a hematologic abnormality in an HIV-positive patient, these disorders may be multifactorial and related to the patient's HIV status or may be independent of the HIV infection. Any attempt to alleviate the abnormality requires the elucidation of the underlying pathogenetic processes.

Anemia

Anemia is defined as a hemoglobin level (Hgb) of <135 g/L in males and <115 g/L in females. When present, a single significant factor can be frequently identified, but often the etiology is multifactorial.

The incidence of anemia in HIV patients increases in tandem with immunologic deterioration through the categories A to C. Thus anemia is present in 3.2 percent of asymptomatic HIV-seropositive patients whose CD4 count is >700 and increases to 20.9 percent if the CD4 count is <249. About 15 percent of patients with persistent generalized adenopathy have anemia, and this incidence increases to between 70 and 90 percent in patients who have progressed to AIDS. Elucidating the mechanisms of anemia requires standard hematologic tests readily available in most laboratories, including the measurement of the mean corpuscular value (MCV) and red cell distribution width, and a careful appraisal of the peripheral blood film. Using these tests, anemias can be classified in terms of (1) cell size (normocytic, macrocytic, or microcytic) or (2) abnormal red blood cell (RBC) morphology (spherocytes, acanthocytes, etc.).

Normocytic Normochromic Anemia

ANEMIA OF CHRONIC DISEASE. Anemia of chronic disease is the commonest form of anemia. In this disorder, on the peripheral blood film the RBC morphology is normal. The reticulocyte count is normal or decreased, and serum iron is low and associated with a normal to low total iron-binding capacity (TIBC). The serum ferritin level is increased, and behaves as an acute phase reactant, its level paralleling the severity of the HIV infection.[1] In the pathogenesis of this type of anemia, iron released from the breakdown of RBCs is returned to the reticuloendothelial system, but then is not released from the stores for use in the formation of RBCs. This can be demonstrated in examination of the bone marrow, which reveals increases in iron by Prussian blue stain in macrophages (tissue iron) but little or no iron in the nucleated RBCs (sideroblasts).

Therapy for this disorder includes the management of any treatable illnesses identified. Erythropoeitin has been shown to be most effective in those with erythropoeitin levels >500 IU/L.[2] It may therefore be of use in selected patients for decreasing the need for blood transfusions and improving quality of life.

INFILTRATIVE MARROW DISORDERS. Infiltrative bone marrow disorders may present as normochromic normocytic anemias. These disorders should be carefully excluded, particularly if the Hgb is <80 g/L or if the Hgb is progressively decreasing. Suspicion is heightened if sidero-blasts or immature granulocytes are present in the peripheral blood film. Disorders commonly infiltrating the marrow include mycobacterial infection (either MAI or *Mycobacterium tuberculosis*), lymphoma, and disseminated fungal infections. The diagnosis can be made in these cases by bone marrow biopsy and appropriate stains for the suspected pathogen. Management consists of appropriate treatment of the pathogen.

Macrocytic Anemia

This type of anemia is characterized by an MCV >100 fl. Various causes of macrocytic anemia must be considered in making a diagnosis. A spurious macrocytosis occurs with cold agglutination, but the agglutinated RBCs are easily identified on the peripheral blood film. Similarly, a brisk reticulocytosis is frequently associated with an elevated MCV, but again, polychromasia is present on the peripheral blood film and can be quantitated by a reticulocyte count. Hypothyroidism, ethanol abuse, and liver disease can also be associated with an increased MCV. The commonest cause of macrocytic anemia in HIV, however, is drug therapy. There has been a great deal of interest in B_{12} and folate metabolism, but these have not been common clinical problems.

DRUGS.   Zidovudine (AZT) is a deoxynucleoside analog with antiretroviral activity. A significant macrocytosis, with an MCV >110 fl, can be demonstrated in about 70 percent of patients on zidovudine after several weeks of therapy. Significant anemia was noted in 34 percent of patients after 6 weeks of therapy.[3] Bone marrow studies reveal megaloblastic changes, hypoplasia, or frank aplasia. The severity of anemia may be reduced by decreasing the dose, stopping the drug for short periods, administering erythropoietin, or judicious use of blood transfusions. The other deoxynucleoside analogs, such as zalcitabine (ddC) and didanosine (ddI), do not appear to have the same propensity to produce anemia.

Megaloblastic Anemia

Serum B_{12} levels are low in approximately 20 percent of patients. In a recent study, vitamin B_{12} malabsorption was not associated with an elevated MCV, hypersegmentation, or megaloblastic marrow, and moreover did not improve with B_{12}.[4] This likely represents a spurious laboratory result. Nonetheless, an abnormal Schilling test has been documented in a group of patients, attributed to decreased absorption in the terminal ileum.[5] Thus in patients with a macrocytic anemia and low B_{12} levels, a Shilling test should be performed, and if abnormal, B_{12} administered.

Myelodysplastic Changes

Myelodysplasia is a term used by hematologists to refer to a group of disorders characterized by one or more pancytopenias and usually hypercellular marrow. The disorder is clonal in nature, associated with chromosomal abnormalities, and frequently evolves into acute leukemia. The FAB classification is a morphologic classification of these disorders.[6] Similar dysplastic morphology can be seen in patients with HIV disease. In the usual clinical situation, these changes are drug related. However, there are a number of cases in which these abnormalities cannot be ascribed to drugs and must reflect the disease process itself. Treatment in these situations is strictly symptomatic and supportive.

Microcytic Normochromic or Hypochromic Anemia

Microcytic anemias by definition are characterized by an MCV <80 fl. Hypochromia can be expressed by RBC indices as a mean corpuscular Hgb <334 g/L. This form of anemia is uncommon in HIV disease. In the context of HIV disease, iron-deficiency anemia or, in some cases, anemia of chronic disease is more likely to be found.

IRON-DEFICIENCY ANEMIA. As iron stores are depleted, the MCV will eventually drop below 80 fl, and the peripheral blood film will reveal initially microcytic, and then with progressive depletion, hypochromic changes. The reticulocyte count is usually normal unless the patient is actively bleeding or is receiving supplemental iron. In uncomplicated cases, the serum iron is low, the TIBC elevated, and the serum ferritin low. To complicate matters, the serum iron may be low because of an underlying disorder, and the ferritin level may be elevated as an acute phase reactant. If iron deficiency is documented, causes specific to AIDS include inflammatory colitis, especially that secondary to CMV infection, Kaposi's sarcoma, lymphoma, and thrombocytopenia, in addition to the causes identified in the general population.

Therapy consists of iron replacement. Slow-release or encapsulated iron preparations should be avoided. The most effective form of parenteral therapy is a liquid iron preparation. With these preparations, however, in addition to the usual side effects of iron therapy, staining of the teeth may occur. This can be offset by brushing with baking soda or by taking the medication through a straw.

Abnormalities of RBC Morphology

IMMUNE HEMOLYTIC ANEMIA.   Although a positive Coombs' test is found in up to 20 percent of AIDS patients, true hemolytic anemia is rare. The cause of the positive Coombs' test in most cases appears to be associated with hypergammaglobulinemia. In the few cases of true hemolytic anemia, the reticulocyte count is elevated, often to a degree sufficient to increase the MCV. A significant number of spherocytes are present in the peripheral blood film. In addition to the Coombs' test, other abnormal laboratory values, such as elevated LDH and decreased haptoglobin, can confirm diagnosis. However, since haptoglobin may also be increased as an acute phase reactant, interpretation of this laboratory value may be difficult. Obtaining a glycosylated HgB level may help resolve this problem because it is a measurement of the time RBCs are in contact with glucose.

Increased indirect serum bilirubin is seen in about 50 percent of patients, but because the test reflects not only RBC breakdown, but also the liver's ability to excrete bilirubin, this test is not particularly sensitive.

Management of immune hemolytic anemia traditionally includes steroids, started at a dose of 1 mg/kg. If hemolysis is fulminant, IV gamma globulin, usually given in a dose of 400 mg/kg for 4 to 5 days, may be useful. Danazol is sometimes effective in ameliorating this disorder, and may decrease the amount of steroids needed. Doses have ranged from 200 mg QID to 50 mg daily. Splenectomy, while an effective therapeutic modality, is the treatment of last resort.

OXIDATIVE HEMOLYSIS.   The normal mechanisms that protect RBCs from oxidative damage stem primarily from the hexose monophosphate shunt. In the presence of strong oxidative drugs, these mechanisms can be overwhelmed. When this occurs, hemoglobin precipitates into Heinz bodies, which are pitted out by the spleen, initiating a hemolytic process. This process is magnified in patients with G6PD deficiency. Morphologic evidence supporting this diagnosis can be found in the peripheral blood film, which reveals, in addition to a reticulocytosis, "bite" and blister cells, evidence of splenic pitting. The drugs that most frequently cause this phenomenon are sulfa drugs and phenazopyridine. Dapsone is a particularly potent oxidative agent that causes mild hemolysis in most patients and a significant hemolytic anemia in a few. High-dose therapy with TMP-SMX (Septra), as used in the treatment of PCP, is a typical clinical scenario in which this disorder can be found.

THROMBOTIC THROMBOCYTOPENIC PURPURA. Thrombotic thrombocytopenic purpura is an uncommon clinical syndrome characterized by fever, neurologic abnormalities, renal dysfunction, microangiopathic hemolytic anemia, and thrombocytopenia. The incidence of this disorder is increased in HIV infections.[7] The etiology of the disorder is still not worked out, but appears to involve damaged vascular endothelium, von Willebrand factor, and platelets. Diagnosis requires a high degree of suspicion and the demonstration of reticulocytosis, microangiopthic RBCs, and megathrombocytes.

This disorder has a high mortality untreated, and once the diagnosis is made the patient should receive fresh frozen plasma immediately. As soon as is technically possible, plasmapheresis should be started, dialysing the patient against plasma or, more optimally, against cryoprecipitate-poor fresh frozen plasma.

Leukopenia

Lymphocytopenia

Infection of CD4 lymphocytes by HIV produces a progressive decline in this cell population, likely related to accelerated apoptosis.[8] However, the absolute peripheral lymphocyte count cannot be used as a diagnostic test, as 15 percent of patients without HIV in hospitals will have lymphocyte counts <1000/mm^3.[9] The correct timing for prophylactic treatment depends on the absolute CD4 count. In the initial phase of the illness the number of CD8 lymphocytes is increased. In the marrow, there is an increase in plasma cells and lymphoid aggregates, likely secondary to dysregulation of lymphopoiesis and frequently associated with an attendant diffuse polyclonal hypergammaglobulinemia.

Neutropenia

Granulocytopenia, defined as a neutrophil count <1500/ml^3, occurs in 10 to 20 percent of patients with AIDS-related complex and 35 to 75 percent of patients with AIDS. Note that in black males of African origin, the lower limit of normal may be as low as 800/ml^3.[10] A number of mechanisms are operative.

INEFFECTIVE MYELOPOIESIS

1. Drug induced.

   - Zidovudine may cause severe neutropenia. Generally the dose of the drug is reduced when the neutrophil count is between 500 and 1000 cells/mm^3. If the neutrophil count is maintained above 500/mm^3, bacterial infections are uncommon. Decreasing the dose or stopping zidovudine is usually followed by prompt recovery.

   - Ganciclovir is another common drug producing neutropenia. Its toxicity is increased when used with zidovudine.[11]

   - Other drugs causing neutropenia include sulfonamides, dihydrofolate reductase inhibitors such as pyrimethamine and trimethoprim, pentamidine, interferon-alpha, antifungal agents, and chemotherapeutic agents.

There are several clinical situations in which cytokines can be used to elevate the neutrophil count. In patients with CMV retinitis, both foscarnet and ganciclovir may produce significant neutropenia, the incidence ranging from 25 to 40 percent. GM-CSF/G-CSF have been demonstrated to be effective in raising the neutrophil count without having any deleterious effects on the retinitis, and are therefore helpful in allowing full-dose therapy to be continued. Another clinical situation encountered involves the maintenance of adequate neutrophil counts during chemotherapy, allowing administration of appropriate doses of chemotherapy. The routine use to support the neutrophil count will likely not be an effective therapeutic modality because so few AIDS patients die of bacterial infections. Currently studies are underway to determine if maintaining a normal neutrophil count with cytokines will decrease admissions to hospital for febrile illnesses.

2. Myelodysplasia. Decreased production of granulocytes can occur independently of drugs. The peripheral blood film may show pseudo-Pelger neutrophils, and the bone marrow, abnormalities both in morphology and maturation of the granulocyte precursors. Treatment here should again be predominantly symptomatic and supportive. In some patients cytokines may be effective in raising the neutrophil count.

3. Immune granulocytopenia. Antibodies commonly can be demonstrated on circulating neutrophils. Like the anti-

bodies demonstrated in the positive Coombs' test, these antibodies generally do not seem to have any physiologic significance. However, cases of immune granulocytopenia have been described as responding to high doses of immunoglobulin G.[12]

Thrombocytopenia

Thrombocytopenia is characterized by a platelet count of <150,000. In general, with fully functional platelets, a patient is hemostatically normal with platelet counts around 50,000. In patients with immune thrombocytopenia, levels ranging from 5 to 10,000 may produce bruising, petechia, submucosal bleeding, and occasionally epistaxis. Rarely are these bleeding episodes of any clinical significance. Such patients may have mild splenomegaly, in contrast to those with acute thrombocytopenia.

Immune thrombocytopenia must be differentiated from other causes of thrombocytopenia that could be present. The diagnosis is made by observing large platelets on the peripheral blood film, and by platelet antibody studies, which usually show immunoglobulin on the platelet surface. Only on rare occasions is a bone marrow test needed to demonstrate an increase in megakaryocytes.

Treatment of thrombocytopenia is controversial, but currently most experts favor no therapy unless significant bleeding is present. Therapy with prednisone (1 mg/kg) may work, but in general the number of patients who respond and the quality of the response is diminished compared to that seen in acute thrombocytopenia. Steroids used in this setting do not appear to produce significant changes in the progression of the HIV disease, or be responsible for an unusual increase in opportunistic fungal infections. High-dose IV gamma globulin has been effective in patients and is usually given in an acute setting where significant bleeding has to be reversed quickly. It is generally administered in a dose of 400 mg/kg for 5 days.[13] Zidovudine will itself improve the platelet count. Studies have shown decreased platelet survival in patients with immune thrombocytopenia.[14] Zidovudine has been found to be an effective method of treating immune thrombocytopenia. Since treating patients with zidovudine does not improve platelet survival, the therapeutic effect must result from the increase in the ability of megakaryocytes to produce platelets. Danazol has been used with some success in doses ranging from 50 to 800 mg/day. Finally, about 66 percent of these patients will respond to splenectomy.

ONCOLOGIC MANIFESTATIONS
Carol Sawka, M.D., F.R.C.P.C.

Kaposi's Sarcoma

The most common tumor diagnosed in AIDS patients is Kaposi's sarcoma (KS).[15] It occurs most frequently in homosexual men, who currently account for 95 percent of cases, however, a growing number of women and children with HIV in Africa also develop KS. The overall incidence of KS as an AIDS-defining illness in homosexuals has decreased since 1981, but the overall lifetime incidence of KS has remained unchanged at 30 to 50 percent of patients with HIV infection. In the early 1980s KS frequently presented as an indolent disease early in the HIV infection associated with a normal CD4 count. However, as the HIV infection progressed in those individuals, the KS became more widespread and symptomatic. Today KS presents more often as a later manifestation of AIDS, is frequently associated with severe immunosuppression (low CD4 counts and previous opportunistic infections), and has a more aggressive course. Although for many patients KS is limited to a few isolated lesions on the skin or mucous membranes, KS can cause more significant morbidity from infiltrative tumor, edema, lymphatic obstruction, organ infiltration, and respiratory compromise in up to 20 percent of cases and recently it has been suggested that up to 30 percent of patients die from complications of KS, although other co-morbidities, such as opportunistic infections, may also be present.[16]

There is wide variation in the clinical presentation of KS. It may just affect the skin with single or multiple lesions. These may be asymptomatic or may be painful or associated with edema. Oral mucus membrane and gastrointestinal lesions frequently develop; although any organ may be involved, the lungs and gastrointestinal tract are the most frequently affected. Cutaneous and oral lesions do not necessarily predict the spread of KS to internal organs.

Pulmonary KS may coincide with lung infection and may be difficult to diagnose. Symptoms include dyspnea, dry cough, and occasional fever. The chest x-ray is frequently abnormal, with nonspecific infiltrates or reticular nodular changes. Bronchoscopy with direct visualization is required for diagnosis and for exclusion of coexistent opportunistic infections. Biopsy is frequently not helpful. Gastrointestinal KS occurs in up to 40 percent of patients with KS on the skin. Many patients are asymptomatic, however, diarrhea, rectal pain, and occult or overt bleeding may occur. Direct visualization of typical mucosal lesions by endoscopy or colonoscopy is required since radiographic studies are usually not helpful. Biopsy often confirms the diagnosis made by direct visualization.

Indications for treatment include cosmetic disfigurement by skin lesions, particularly those on the face or those associated with significant edema, as well as pain, obstruction, particularly of the oropharynx, and visceral involvement, particularly of the pulmonary system.

Wherever possible local treatment is delivered. This may include use of cosmetics, cryotherapy with liquid nitrogen, and laser treatment. Radiation therapy may produce improvement in up to 80 percent of cases and is particularly useful in controlling pain and edema. Intralesional chemotherapy with vinblastine and interferon-alpha has been used for oral lesions where radiation therapy may cause severe mucositis.

Systemic therapy is used when necessary to control the general effects of disease. Interferon-alpha with concurrent zidovudine is useful if the immune function is relatively well preserved with a CD4 count of >200 and where there is not history of previous opportunistic infections; however, due to the late presentation of KS in recent years, most patients are not suitable for interferon-alpha and instead chemotherapy is recommended. Relatively indolent disease may be treated with a single chemotherapeutic agent such as vinblastine. Combination therapy with doxorubicin, bleomycin, and vincristine results in more rapid resolution of symptoms, with partial responses in up to 70 percent of cases.

Although local and systemic therapy are both very useful in controlling symptoms their impact on overall survival has not been demonstrated in randomized controlled trials.

Patients should be referred to an oncologist when treatment for KS is indicated.

Non-Hodgkin's Lymphoma

Non-Hodgkin's lymphoma (NHL) is an AIDS-defining event in 3 percent of AIDS patients, but accounts for 12 to

16 percent of all AIDS-related deaths.[17] AIDS-related NHL tends to occur with more advanced HIV disease with described associated factors of previous KS, previous opportunistic infection, and low neutrophil count. Six to eight years after the onset of HIV infection the risk of lymphoma increases 100-fold and approximates 1 percent per year following a diagnosis of AIDS. Although prolonged zidovudine therapy has been epidemiologically linked to an increased risk of lymphoma, this does not appear to be causative, but rather relates to prolonged survival times with HIV in the current AIDS era. As the CD4 count declines to <50 to 100, the incidence of lymphoma increases and primary brain lymphoma is frequently seen with very low CD4 counts.

AIDS-related NHL is a high-grade B-cell-phenotype lymphoma, usually with extranodal presentation, often involving the gastrointestinal tract and brain. Diagnosis is by biopsy. Symptoms such as fever, night sweats, and weight loss are common. CNS tumors count for 10 to 20 percent of lymphomas in AIDS patients and are characterized by seizures, focal neurologic deficits, and headache. The CT scan appears nonspecific (i.e., single or multiple low-density contrast-enhancing mass lesions with surrounding edema). AIDS-related NHL has an aggressive clinical course, with a median survival of 2.8 months for CNS and 6.0 months for systemic lymphoma. A history of AIDS, a CD4 count of ≤200, a Karnofsky performance of <70 percent, and stage IV disease, especially with bone marrow involvement, influence survival times, with 11- to 12-month median survivals seen in the absence of all of these features and only 4-month survivals with one or more of these features.

Optimal treatment is with chemotherapy regardless of stage at presentation. This achieves a 50 percent complete remission rate and a 6-month average survival. Mortality is due to opportunistic infections in half of the cases and lymphoma in the other half. Low-dose chemotherapy regimens appear to decrease the rate of opportunistic infections while maintaining survival rates. The concept of dose intensity was recently tested in one randomized trial.[18] The use of a hematopoietic growth factor, GM-CSF, with full-dose chemotherapy did not improve complete response rates, response durations, or survival times compared with a low-dose version of the same chemotherapy regimen without growth factor support. Several clinical trials of novel drugs or schedules of administrations, such as prolonged IV infusion of drugs, have been conducted, with no clearly superior results to date. Clinical trials are ongoing. Radiation therapy for CNS lymphoma can ameliorate symptoms, but does not improve survival times.

References

HEMATOLOGIC MANIFESTATIONS

1. Gupta S, Inman A, Licorish K. Serum ferritin in acquired immune deficiency syndrome. J Clin Lab Immunol 1986; 20:11.
2. Henry DH, Gildon NB, et al. Recombinant human erythropoietin in the treatment of anemia associated with human immunodeficiency virus (HIV) infection and zidovudine therapy. Ann Intern Med 1992; 117:739.
3. Richman DD, Fischl MA, Grieco MH. The toxicity of azidothymidine in the treatment of patients with AIDS and AIDS-related complex. N Engl J Med 1987; 317:192.
4. Aboulafia DM, Mitsuyasu RT. Hematological abnormalities in AIDS. Hematol Oncol Clin North Am 1991; 5:195.
5. Harriman G, Smith P, Horne M. Vitamin B_{12} malabsorption in patients with acquired immunodeficiency syndrome. Arch Intern Med 1989; 149:2039.
6. Bennett JM, Catovsky D, et al. Proposals for the classification of the myelodysplastic syndromes. Br J Haematol 1982; 51:189.
7. Nair J, Bellevue R, Bertoni M. Thrombotic thromboctopenic purpura in patients with the acquired immunodeficiency syndrome-related complex. Ann Intern Med 1988; 109:209.
8. Oyaizu N, McCloskey TW, Coronesi N. Accelerated apoptosis in peripheral blood mononuclear cells from human immunodeficiency type-1 infected patients. Blood 1993; 82:3392.
9. Boyko WJ, Schecter MT, Constance P. Limited usefulness of lymphocytopenia in screening for AIDS in a hospital population. Can Med Assoc J 1985; 133:293.
10. Shaper AG, Lewis P. Genetic neutropenia in people of African origin. Lancet 1971; 2:1021.
11. Hochster H, Dieterich D, Bozzette S. Toxicity of combined ganciclovir and zidovudine for cytomegalovirus disease associated with AIDS. Ann Intern Med 1990; 113:111.
12. Salama A, Lohmeyer J, Seeger W. High dose IgG for neuropenic patients with acquired immunodeficiency syndrome. Ann Hematol 1991; 63:77.
13. Perret B, Baumgartner C. Workshop on immunotherapy of lymphoproliferative syndromes, mainly AIDS-related complex and AIDS. Vox Sang 1986; 52:1.
14. Bei-Ali Z, Dufour V, Najean Y. Platelet kinetics in human immunodeficiency induced thrombocytopenia. Am J Hematol 1987; 26:299.

ONCOLOGIC MANIFESTATIONS

15. Buckbinder A, Freidman-Kiene, AE. Clinical aspects of Kaposi sarcoma. *Curr Opin Oncol* 1992; 4:867-74.
16. Mitsuyasu RT. The pathogenesis and treatment of AIDS related Kaposi sarcoma. Educational Book from the 31st Annual Meeting of the American Society of Clinical Oncology, p. 160.

17. Levine AM. AIDS-related malignancies: The emerging epidemic (review): J Nat Cancer Instit 1993; 85:1382.
18. Kaplan L, Straus D, Test M, et al. Randomized trial of standard dose m BACOP with G-MCSF versus reduced dose m BACOD for systemic HIV associated lymphoma: ACTG 142. Proc Am Soc Clin Oncol 1995; 14:288.

▬ RENAL MANIFESTATIONS

Gavril Hercz, M.D., F.R.C.P.C.

As the number of HIV-infected patients grows, an increasing number of renal syndromes are being recognized, affecting 2 to 10 percent of patients. These syndromes provide a challenge in finding specific therapies that will prolong renal survival or reverse the renal insufficiency already sustained. The presence of previous renal insufficiency also presents a challenge in terms of the need to modify drug type and dosage. Aside from numerous biochemical abnormalities, various renal parenchymal disorders resulting in clinical disease have been reported. The major issues to be dealt with include the following:

1. Fluid, electrolyte, and acid–base disturbances.

2. Renal parenchymal disorders:

   - Acute tubular necrosis.

   - HIV-associated nephropathy.

   - Miscellaneous glomerular, vascular, and tubulointerstitial disorders.

3. Dialysis.

FLUID, ELECTROLYTE, AND ACID–BASE DISTURBANCES

Hyponatremia

Hyponatremia has been found to occur in 50 percent of hospitalized AIDS/AIDS-related complex (ARC) patients. It is a poor prognostic indicator, with 30 percent of patients dying during the admission, twice the mortality rate of admitted normonatremic patients. The etiology of hyponatremia is as follows:

1. *Hypovolemic* causes, diagnosed clinically by evaluation of the patient's volume status as well as the presence of low urinary sodium (<15 mmol/L) secondary to

   - gastrointestinal fluid losses with or without replacement of losses with hypotonic solutions (e.g., D_5W).
   - adrenocortical insufficiency (5 percent). This is usually seen with adrenalitis caused by infection with CMV, MAC, or HIV itself. It is also seen with adrenal hemorrhage and infiltrative Kaposi's sarcoma. Patients may have associated hyperkalemia, nonanion gap metabolic acidosis, hypovolemia, or renal sodium wasting.

2. *Normovolemic* causes, due to the syndrome of inappropriate antidiuretic hormone secretion secondary to

   - *P. carinii* or other forms of pneumonitis.
   - CNS infection.
   - malignancy.

3. *Hypervolemic* causes, mainly due to acute renal failure.

Hyperkalemia and Hypokalemia

Hyperkalemia is found in 15 to 20 percent of hospitalized patients. The causes include the following:

1. Hyporeninemic hypoaldosteronism, which may respond to treatment with fludrocortisone 0.1 to 0.2 mg/day.
2. Adrenocortical insufficiency (see Hyponatremia).
3. Diabetes mellitus developing from pentamidine-induced pancreatic islet cell dysfunction.
4. Acute renal failure.
5. Drugs, including pentamidine (blocks distal potassium secretion) and high-dose trimethoprim (acts as potassium-sparing diuretic).

Hypokalemia is caused by several factors:

1. Severe diarrhea.
2. Vomiting with subsequent urinary losses of potassium.
3. Gentamicin- or amphotericin B-induced renal losses.

Metabolic Alkalosis

Causes include hypokalemia and upper gastrointestinal tract fluid losses.

Metabolic Acidosis

1. Increased anion gap:

- Lactic acidosis
- Sepsis.
- Idiopathic form associated with abnormal lactate metabolism.
- Renal failure.

2. Normal anion gap:

- Diarrhea
- Adrenocortical insufficiency (see Hyponatremia).
- Distal renal tubular acidosis (drug-induced interstitial nephritis).

Hypercalcemia

1. Elevated levels of 1-25 dihydroxycholecalciferol secondary to infection with tuberculosis or B-cell lymphoma. This responds to restriction of oral calcium intake, elimination of vitamin D supplements, avoidance of sun exposure, and administration of low-dose prednisone (10 to 30 mg/day).
2. Elevated PTHrP associated with T-cell lymphoma and disseminated CMV infection.

Hypomagnesemia

1. Diarrhea.
2. Drugs: amphotericin B, pentamidine.

RENAL PARENCHYMAL DISORDERS

Acute Tubular Necrosis

Given the frequency of sepsis in admitted patients in association with hypotension and exposure to multiple nephrotoxic agents, it is not surprising that both oliguric and nonoliguric acute tubular necrosis (ATN) are frequently seen. The patients usually recover but may require dialytic support temporarily. In many cases, conservative therapy with appropriate fluid management and withdrawal of the toxic agent results in quick recovery.

ATN has two major causes:

1. Ischemia resulting from sepsis, or blood or fluid loss.

2. Nephrotoxins, including

- Gentamicin.

- Pentamidine, which results in ATN in 25 percent of patients given the drug. It has also been noted with the nebulized form. There is increased risk if the patient is volume contracted or prescribed other potential nephrotoxins. ATN resolves over several weeks. Once the patient recovers, pentamidine should be avoided in the future since recurrent renal insufficiency may occur. Hyperkalemia, urinary magnesium wasting, and hypocalcemia have also been noted with pentamidine.

- Acyclovir.

- Amphotericin B.

- Foscarnet: during its use two-thirds of patients have a detectable rise in serum creatinine occurring after 6 to 15 days of therapy and 10 to 15 percent eventually require temporary dialysis. Volume repletion with 2.5 L/day, started the night before therapy and continued through the therapy period, may reduce the risk of ATN. As the drug is renally excreted, the dose should be modified in renal insufficiency.

- Rhabdomyolysis secondary to HIV or zidovudine therapy: when associated with volume contraction, acute renal failure may result.

HIV-Associated Nephropathy

First described in 1984, this lesion is characterized by the appearance of heavy proteinuria, rapidly progressive renal insufficiency, and nephrotic syndrome. Clinically it occurs in 2 to 10 percent of HIV-infected patients and accounts for 80 percent of chronic renal failure in AIDS patients. It occurs more commonly in males and blacks, and less commonly in gay white men. It has also been reported in HIV-infected children. Half the patients may be asymptomatic carriers or those with ARC; thus HIV-associated nephropathy may predate clinical AIDS by months/years. Patients present with the nephrotic syndrome (edema, heavy proteinuria, and hypoalbuminemia). Hyperlipidemia is less commonly seen as compared to non-HIV-infected patients with the nephrotic syndrome. On urinalysis, there is a lack of cellular elements. Renal ultrasound demonstrates large echogenic kidneys. Pathologically, collapsing focal and segmental glomerulosclerosis is seen, with severe tubulointerstitial disease. On electron microscopy, tubuloreticular structures are noted in the glomerular endothelial cells. Most patients experience rapidly progressive, irreversible azotemia, reaching dialysis within 4 to 6 months of diagnosis. There is no known therapy but survival is short even when dialysis is initiated. Zidovudine administration may slow progression of disease, although many causes of HIV-associated nephropathy develop in individuals already on zidovudine or didanosine. Also, steroids may be beneficial but one has to weigh the possible side effects. The role of cyclosporin is currently being explored.

Miscellaneous Lesions

1. Acute proliferative postinfectious glomerulonephritis may be seen with significant IgA or IgG deposits. On urinalysis, an active urinary sediment is noted with RBCs and cellular casts. Spontaneous remission may occur in some patients, while others have responded to corticosteroid/cytotoxic agent combinations.

2. Membranous glomerulonephritis secondary to hepatitis B infection or syphilis.

3. Interstitial nephritis, seen with

   - drug allergy (TMP-SMX, phenytoin).
   - opportunistic infections.
   - calcification (amphotericin B).

These patients may present with fever, oliguria, elevated serum creatinine, mild proteinuria, and WBCs or white cell casts on urinalysis.

4. Invasion of renal parenchyma with lymphoma, Kaposi's sarcoma.

5. Amyloidosis secondary to subcutaneous narcotic injection.

6. Hemolytic uremic syndrome/thrombotic thrombocytopenic purpura is increasingly recognized. It is related to endothelial cell injury by a variety of factors. Clinically, it presents with fever, fluctuating neurologic signs, renal dysfunction, microangiopathic hemolytic anemia, and thrombocytopenia. LDH levels are elevated and schistocytes are seen on peripheral smear. Patients respond to plasma exchange. On a long-term basis it has a poor prognosis, with survival of less than 2 years after the diagnosis is made.

7. IgA nephropathy is also increasingly being reported. It may present with gross hematuria (40 to 50 percent), microscopic hematuria (30 to 40 percent), or acute glomerulonephritis (10 percent). Very minimal proteinuria is detected as compared to HIV-associated nephropathy. Electron microscopy reveals the same tubuloreticular structures noted in endothelial cells as seen with HIV-associated nephropathy. In postmortem studies approximately 8 percent of HIV-infected patients had IgA deposits in their kidneys, which in the majority of patients was not clinically detected antemortem.

8. Minimal-change disease.

9. Diffuse mesangial proliferative glomerulonephritis, seen in pediatric patients presenting with nephrotic syndrome.

10. Membranoproliferative glomerulonephritis, type I.

DIALYSIS

Chronic renal insufficiency is almost always caused by HIV-associated nephropathy. Although the incidence of end-stage renal disease varies from 1 to 5.7 percent of all AIDS patients, depending on the study population, the percentage actually started on dialysis varies from 0.3 to 4.1 percent. Peritoneal dialysis and hemodialysis are equally efficacious. The prognosis once on dialysis varies: patients with AIDS survive only 9 months, as compared to patients with ARC or asymptomatic carriers, who survive for 1 to 2 years. The usual cause of death is a severe cachexia that is unresponsive to hyperalimentation.

Suggested Readings

1. Rao TKS. Clinical features of human immunodeficiency virus associated nephropathy. Kidney Int 1991; 40: S13–8.
2. Glassock RJ, Cohen AH, Danovitch G, Parsa KP. Human immunodeficiency virus (HIV) infection and the kidney. Ann Intern Med 1990; 112: 35–50.
3. Seney FD, Jr, Burns DK, Silva F. Acquired immunodeficiency syndrome and the kidney. Am J Kidney Dis 1990; 16: 1–13.
4. Tang WW, Kaptein EM, Feinstein EI, Massry SG. Hyponatremia in hospitalized patients with acquired immunodeficiency syndrome (AIDS) and the AIDS-related complex. Am J Med 1993; 94: 169–4.
5. Leaf AN, Lanbestein LJ, Raphael B et al. Thrombotic thrombocytopenic purpura associated with human immunodeficiency virus type I (HIV-1) infection. Ann Intern Med 1988; 109: 194–7.

DERMATOLOGIC MANIFESTATIONS
Benjamin K. Fisher, M.D., F.R.C.P.C.

With time, skin conditions will affect all individuals with HIV infection. Diagnosing these conditions may be harder than in otherwise healthy patients because of the wide spectrum of skin lesions, and their many atypical presentations.

INFECTIONS

Shingles (herpes zoster virus infection) frequently develops in both early and advanced HIV disease; it is usually confined to one or more dermatomes, but is occasionally widespread. Acyclovir is recommended by most authorities, despite the absence of randomized trials confirming its benefits in this disease. Any ulcer around the anus, penis, mouth, or digits should be attributed to herpes simplex; if a diagnosis cannot be made clinically, either acyclovir should be given empirically or tissue/cells obtained for culture (or Tzanck preparation). Where available, a scraping from the base of a blister can be checked for herpes simplex or zoster using monoclonal antibodies, and the result reported within 2 hours. Molluscum contagiosum, caused by a pox virus, is a very common infection characterized by shiny skin-colored umbilicated papules that appear on the face, trunk, or genitals. The papules increase rapidly in size and number. Cryotherapy, electrocautery, and other destructive modalities usually provide only temporary relief, and recurrence is common. Warts on the fingers, hands, and feet, and particularly in the perianal area and on the genitals, are difficult to treat and tend to recur after treatment with any modality.

The most prevalent bacterial pathogens in AIDS are *Staphylococcus aureus* and streptococci, usually presenting as pruritic folliculitis or impetigo. Cephalosporins and other antibiotics are usually effective, although abscesses also require incision and drainage. Syphilis (in homosexual men) and disseminated mycobacterial infections are other not-to-be-missed but treatable infectious lesions in AIDS.

Hairy leukoplakia is an abnormal, white, corrugated thickening of the lateral tongue; unlike oral candidiasis, the lesions of this process are difficult to scrape off. It occurs almost exclusively in HIV infection, and may predict progression to AIDS. Epstein–Barr virus can be isolated from the lesions, sometimes together with papilloma virus.

Because hairy leukoplakia is rarely painful, treatment is usually not necessary, although some benefit has been recorded by using oral descyclovir (which is converted to acyclovir in vivo), or from sucking clotrimazole lozenges.

Another dermatologic infection unique to HIV is bacillary angiomatosis, which usually appears as friable red smooth nodules, ulcers, plaques, or papules. DNA hybridization techniques suggest the causative pathogen is closely related to the agent responsible for cat-scratch fever, *Rochalimaea quintana* or *R. henselae*. Recent work has implicated the *Bartonella bacillus*. Diagnosis, by biopsy, is necessary because erythromycin and tetracycline have been found to control this potentially fatal condition.

Tinea cruris, tinea pedis, and tinea versicolor are frequent in early and late HIV infection, often present atypically, and resist standard treatments.

NEOPLASTIC DISEASES

The classical Kaposi's sarcoma lesion is a violaceous nodule or plaque on the lower limbs, but in HIV disease it can be red, blue, or brown and may present as a macule, papule, or plaque virtually anywhere on the skin, mucosae, or internal organs. There is no correlation between the extent of cutaneous involvement and visceral lesions. The natural history is unpredictable: usually there is progression but there may be no change for months to years, followed by acceleration with the sudden emergence of crops of new lesions, and/or confluence of old ones. Kaposi's sarcoma develops primarily in homosexual men. Differential diagnosis includes hemangioma, pyogenic granuloma, lichen planus, dermatofibroma, ecchymosis, nevus, and melanoma. Punch biopsy is recommended in all but characteristic and recognizable cases. Treatment is necessary only if clinical problems develop. Management includes radiation, chemotherapy, excision of small tumors, and intralesional vinblastine injections.

There have been several reports of basal and squamous cell cancers in HIV disease, especially in the mouth and anorectum. Lymphomas may present as nodules or papules on the skin.

PAPULOSQUAMOUS DISORDERS

Seborrheic dermatitis is found in 46 percent of AIDS patients, compared to 5 percent in the general population. It is characterized by erythematous, greasy-yellow scaly plaques, especially in the scalp, eyebrows, ears, center of the face, groin, axillae, and chest. In AIDS it can also involve the trunk and extremities, and tends to be severe and resistant to topical corticosteroids. Topical ketoconazole is reportedly sometimes helpful. The condition may precede all other signs of HIV infection by months to years.

The prevalence of psoriasis does not increase with HIV, but this condition and HIV infection tend to develop concurrently. In other cases, an exacerbation of chronic psoriasis occurs when HIV infection develops. Methotrexate, which has proved helpful in refractory psoriasis, is contraindicated in AIDS because it is said to cause leukopenia, infection, and death in this disease.

Reiter syndrome, a triad of urethritis, conjunctivitis, and arthritis, is also associated with keratotic papules and pustules on the palms and soles (keratoderma blennorhagicum), oral ulcers, and circinate balanitis. These skin lesions are very similar to psoriasis. Recent reports demonstrate an increase in the prevalence of Reiter syndrome in HIV infection.

OTHER SKIN CONDITIONS

Hypersensitivity rashes reportedly develop in up to 50 percent of HIV-infected patients given TMP-SMX. Characteristically, the rash appears as a diffuse maculopapular eruption accompanied by fever. Foscarnet may cause nonhealing erosions on the genitals. Insect bite reactions tend to be florid in AIDS, often defying both diagnosis and treatment. Telangiectasias may be associated with the complete spectrum of HIV disease, typically appearing across the upper chest. Itchy papular eruptions may be secondary to folliculitis, scabies, or eosinophilic pustular psoriasis, or occur as a primary condition in AIDS.

The exanthem of acute HIV infection develops 1 to 3 weeks after viral exposure. Usually it is an asymptomatic, fine, symmetrical, erythematous morbilliform eruption involving the trunk and arms.

Thinning and premature graying of the hair are common.

Suggested Readings

Warner LC, Fisher BK. Cutaneous manifestations of the acquired immunodeficiency syndrome. Int J Dermatol 1986;25:337–50.
Fisher BK, Warner LC. Cutaneous manifestations of the acquired immunodeficiency syndrome. Update 1987. Int J Dermatol 1987;26:615–30.

■■■ OPPORTUNISTIC INFECTIONS

CANDIDA

Mary Fanning, M.D., Ph.D., F.R.C.P.C., F.A.C.P.

Candida infections affect mainly the oropharynx (thrush) and esophagus, and present when the immune system is still relatively intact, with CD4 counts around 400. But a diagnosis of candidiasis denotes an increased likelihood of progression to an AIDS-defining illness. *Candida* esophagitis is an AIDS-defining illness that occurs with CD4 counts <200.

Oral Candidiasis

Oral candidiasis can present in several ways, the most common being pseudomembranous candidiasis, with typical white plaques on the oral mucous membranes that can be easily scraped off, leaving an erythematous or hemorrhagic base. Less common forms include atrophic candidiasis, with smooth red patches on the hard or soft palate, and candidal leukoplakia or hyperkeratosis, in which white lesions appear on the buccal mucosa, tongue, and hard palate. These lesions cannot be scraped off but respond slowly to prolonged antifungal therapy. Patients may be completely asymptomatic or experience pain in the mouth, burning on eating or drinking certain foods, and a sore throat. Diagnosis is made clinically and supported by a smear from the lesion taken for Gram stain or potassium hydroxide preparation.

Candidal Esophagitis

Candidal esophagitis commonly presents together with oral candidiasis, frequently leading to dysphagia, and less frequently to odynophagia and retrosternal esophageal pain. The diagnosis can be confirmed by endoscopy and biopsy of the esophageal mucosa.

Treatment

Oral candidiasis usually responds readily to topical treatment with antifungal agents for 1 to 2 weeks:

- Nystatin oral suspension 500,000 units/QID swish and swallow.

- Nystatin oral pastilles, 200,000 U five times daily.
- Clotrimazole oral troches 10 mg five times daily.

Systemic agents may be necessary in severe cases or those that fail to improve with topical treatment. These include

- Ketoconazole 200 mg BID.
- Fluconazole 200 mg on the first day, then 100 mg daily.
- Itraconazole 200 mg daily.

Oral candida may relapse rapidly or recur frequently, calling for prolonged therapy with topical agents, ketoconazole 200 mg daily or fluconazole 100 mg three times weekly, or 50 mg daily. There is a recent upswing in clinically resistant candida, most often seen after prolonged suppressive therapy and associated with low CD4 counts. Therefore, needless suppressive therapy is best avoided.

Candidal esophagitis requires systemic therapy for 1 to 3 weeks with any of the following:

- Fluconazole 200 mg first day then 100 mg daily.
- Ketoconazole 200 mg BID.
- Itraconazole 200 mg daily.

Fluconazole has been shown more effective in achieving clinical and endoscopic cure. Maintenance therapy may be needed and should be given as fluconazole 100 mg weekly or 50 mg daily.

For clinically unresponsive cases, topical agents may be coadministered. However, if symptoms persist or are severe, IV amphotericin B 0.3 mg/kg/day for 1 week may be administered.

Other medications currently under investigation include amphotericin lozenges, which may be used as an alternative treatment for resistant cases. In some severe and protracted cases, ultimately no agent or combination of agents is effective.

Suggested Readings

Drugs for AIDS and associated infections. Med Lett 1995; 37: 87–94.

Gazzard BG, Smith D. Oral candidosis in HIV-infected patients. Br J Clin Pract 1991; Suppl. 71: 102–8.

Just-Nubling G, Gentschew G, Meisner K, et al. Fluconazole prophylaxis of recurrent oral candidiasis in HIV positive patients. Eur J Clin Microbiol Infect Dis 1991; 10: 917-21.

Laine L, Dretler RH, Contreas CN, et al. Fluconazole compared with ketoconazole for the treatment of Candida esophagitis in AIDS. Ann Intern Med 1992; 117: 655–60.

■ CRYPTOCOCCAL MENINGITIS
Krystyna Ostrowska, M.D., F.R.C.P.C.

Cryptococcal meningitis, caused by a yeast, *Cryptococcus neoformans,* is the most common form of cryptococcosis in AIDS patients, seen when CD4 cell counts go <100.

Care givers should be on the alert for concurrent spread to extraneural sites (blood, lung, genitourinary tract, bone marrow). The clinical picture is an indolent, nonspecific, slowly progressing illness with malaise, fatigue, loss of appetite, mild headache, and intermittent fevers. Fever and headache occur in 60 to 80 percent of patients. Stiff neck, photophobia, nausea, altered mental status, and seizures are far less frequent.

Diagnosis requires demonstration of cryptococcal antigen (CRAG) in serum and cerebrospinal fluid (CSF) and/or positive India Ink stain of CSF, confirmed by a culture of cryptococcus from CSF and/or serum. CSF protein, glucose, and cell count can be normal in many cases, and therefore are not reliable in excluding the condition.

Treatment is with amphotericin B (IV) or, for milder cases, fluconazole (PO), with an option of adding 5-flucytosine to either regimen in the first 2 to 3 weeks of therapy. Beyond this period flucytosine tends to be poorly tolerated because of bone marrow suppression.

Following initial therapy, long-term suppression is continued with either amphotericin B or fluconazole.

The response to therapy can be monitored by improved bclinical condition, supported by a repeat CSF culture for fungus.

Predictors of Poor Outcome

1. On initial presentation:

   - Decreased level of consciousness.
   - Serum sodium <135 mg/dl.
   - High CSF opening pressure.
   - Positive India Ink stain.
   - CSF CRAG >1:1054.
   - CSF WBC <20.
   - Extraneural site.

2. Following primary treatment (at 10 weeks):

- CSF CRAG >1:8.
- Persistently positive cultures from serum or CSF.

Treatment

FIRST CHOICE.   Amphotericin B (IV) 0.7 mg/kg/day
± 5-flucytosine (PO) 100 to 150 mg/kg/day, monitoring peak
levels (25 to 100 μg/ml) for the first 2 to 3 weeks; then
fluconazole (PO) 400 mg daily to complete 8 to 10 weeks;
then maintenance therapy (see below).

SECOND CHOICE.   In mild cases (PO or IV), fluconazole 400 mg/day ± 5-flucytosine 100 to 150 mg/kg/day
for the first 2 to 3 weeks; then fluconazole 400 mg/day to
complete 8 to 10 weeks; then maintenance therapy (see
below).

Chronic Maintenance

Fluconazole (PO) 200 mg/day or amphotericin B 1 mg/kg
two to three times weekly.

Mild cases are defined by the presence of all of the
following:

- Normal level of consciousness or presentation.
- Normal CSF opening pressure.
- Negative India Ink stain of CSF.
- CSF CRAG <1:32.
- No extraneural sites.

Fluconazole may be considered in mild cases if there are
no contraindications to the use of the drug.

Indications for Admission

- Decreased level of consciousness.
- Generalized seizures or status epilepticus.
- Need for IV therapy (see Predictors of Poor Outcome).
- Severe neurologic deficit with inability to cope at home.
- Intolerance of oral medications (PO fluconazole).

Follow-up

For primary therapy initiated on an outpatient basis or
follow-up after hospital discharge:

- Visits q2 weeks for 8 to 10 weeks, then monthly.

- Routine neurologic assessment during the initial 2 months of therapy.
- Repeated CSF culture for fungus at 10 weeks, before lowering to the maintenance dose.

Routine serum or CSF CRAG gives no predictive clues regarding the response to initial therapy or relapse of previously suppressed infection.

Clinical observation of new or recurrent symptoms compatible with cryptococcal meningitis is the best predictor of relapse. If suspected, lumbar puncture should be done and evaluated as outlined earlier in this chapter.

Suggested Readings

AIDS Management Conference. Fort Lauderdale, FL, March 11–14, 1993.

Rachlis AR. Grand Rounds in Infectious Diseases. Sept./Oct. 1991, pp. 15–18.

Saag MS, et al. Comparison of amphotericin B with fluconazole in the treatment of acute AIDS-associated cryptococcal meningitis. N Engl J Med 1992;326, 83–9.

CYTOMEGALOVIRUS

Alice Tseng, Pharm.D.

Tong Yeung, M.D., B.B.S., M.R.C.P.(U.K.), F.C.C.P.

Mary Fanning, M.D., Ph.D., F.R.C.P.C., F.A.C.P.

Disease secondary to infection with cytomegalovirus (CMV) is extremely common in AIDS patients. CMV, a member of the herpes virus family, is acquired throughout life; by the age of 50 years, approximately 50 percent of the general population is CMV seropositive. The incidence of seropositivity may be even higher in certain groups of HIV-infected patients. It is recommended that all HIV-positive individuals be screened for the presence of CMV antibody during initial workup; those who are CMV seronegative should be screened yearly.

In addition, if a blood transfusion is ever required, immunocompromised people who are CMV seronegative should be provided with CMV-negative blood if available, or with unscreened blood that has been filtered with a leukocyte removal filter. This is strongly supported by published literature, primarily in bone marrow transplant recipients. In terms of people who are already CMV seropositive, there is currently no evidence to support the use of CMV-seronegative blood. The literature suggests that in this subpopulation, routine provision of unscreened blood does not seem to adversely affect clinical outcome or disease progression.

In HIV-infected patients, CMV disease is due to reactivation of the latent virus in a previously infected host. Usually, symptomatic CMV disease occurs once CD4 counts fall to <100. Any organ may be affected by CMV, and the clinical manifestations are protean. Common diseases caused by CMV include chorioretinitis, esophagitis, colitis, pneumonia, encephalitis, neuropathy, biliary tract disease (cholangitis), hepatitis, and adrenalitis.

Not all patients with blood, urine, or tissue cultures positive for CMV have clinical symptoms of the infection, and diagnosis of disease caused by CMV should be made by tissue biopsy with histologic evidence of virus-mediated damage (i.e., inclusion cells). Detection of CMV antigen or nucleic acid in tissues is another method for establishing that CMV is actually causing infection. If viral culture is positive for CMV and no other pathogen is identified, the virus may be taken as the cause of illness, and a therapeutic trial of antiviral therapy may be warranted.

Acyclovir is not effective against CMV. Currently available effective antivirals are ganciclovir and foscarnet. These agents have potent anti-CMV activity, but are also associated with serious toxicity. Traditionally, both of these agents have only been available as IV therapy. Since most patients require prolonged therapy (i.e., with CMV retinitis, evidence supports life-long therapy to prevent or delay disease progression), insertion of a permanent indwelling central line (e.g., Hickman or Port-a-Cath) is often necessary. Requirement for daily infusions is associated with many drawbacks, including risk of line infection or sepsis, decreased quality of life, inconvenience, and great expense. Recently, new formulations of ganciclovir have been developed, allowing administration either orally or intraocularly via sustained-release implants. These options are discussed in further detail later in this chapter.

Disease Manifestations

Chorioretinitis

CMV retinitis is the most common ocular manifestation in HIV patients, and is observed in about 25 percent of AIDS patients. Patients usually present with complaints of visual blurring, decreased visual acuity, "floaters," or unilateral visual field loss. There are usually no symptoms of ocular pain or photophobia. CMV retinitis is typically characterized by findings of large, creamy to yellowish-white granular areas with perivascular exudates and hemorrhages (referred to as a "cottage cheese and ketchup appearance") and retinal atrophy on fundoscopic examination. There is usually minimal vitreous and anterior chamber inflammation. CMV retinitis must be distinguished from commonly occurring "cotton wool spots," which are usually asymptomatic and appear as small, fluffy white lesions with indistinct margins, without exudate or hemorrhage.

If left untreated, the disease is progressive in 90 percent of patients. Once the fovea of the retina becomes involved, retinal detachment and/or blindness may occur. Progression of CMV retinitis may be rapid; thus, diagnosed patients should be started on appropriate therapy as soon as possible, especially if the detected lesion is considered to be immediately sight-threatening (i.e., a "zone 1" retinal lesion, located within 1500 μM of the optic disc or within 3000 μM of the fovea).

Improvement is seen in approximately 80 to 90 percent of patients treated with ganciclovir or foscarnet. Because these agents are virustatic, and because of HIV patients' impaired immunity, life-long maintenance therapy is essential.

Gastrointestinal Infection

ESOPHAGITIS.   Esophagitis occurs in approximately 10 percent of AIDS patients who develop CMV disease. Odynophagia is more commonly encountered with CMV esophagitis than in patients with candidal esophagitis. Other symptoms include dysphagia, epigastric pain, and weight loss. Endoscopic appearance varies from discrete single ulcers to extremely large, shallow, superficial ulcerations. Approximately 80 percent of patients show clinical improvement when treated with ganciclovir or foscarnet.

COLITIS.   Diarrhea, weight loss, anorexia, and fever afflict at least 5 to 10 percent of AIDS patients. Colonoscopy reveals diffuse submucosal hemorrhages and diffuse mucosal ulcerations. Indeed, the mucosa may look normal in 10 percent of those with histologic evidence of CMV colitis.

Patients with symptomatic enterocolitis who have no other pathogens detected by endoscopy, histology, or culture, but have CMV detected by these methods may benefit from treatment with either IV ganciclovir or foscarnet. It is uncertain whether maintenance therapy is beneficial in prolonging time to disease progression or preventing the development of CMV disease in other end organs. Currently, there is an ongoing trial to evaluate the role of oral ganciclovir as maintenance therapy for CMV enterocolitis (further information can be obtained from the Syntex Study Centre: phone 1-800-569-4630, fax 1-812-474-7956).

Pneumonia

CMV is commonly isolated from pulmonary secretions or lung tissue of AIDS patients with pneumonia who undergo bronchoscopy, but a true pathogenic role for the virus in AIDS is not apparent. The diagnosis of CMV pneumonia depends not only on a positive CMV culture from lung tissue or pulmonary secretions, but also on the presence of pathognomonic cells with inclusion bodies, CMV antigen or nucleic acid in tissue, and the absence of other pathogenic organisms.

CMV causes an interstitital pneumonia in which patients often complain of slowly progressive shortness of breath, dyspnea on exertion, and a dry, nonproductive cough. Fever, tachycardia, and tachypnea are commonly present. Chest signs are minimal. Chest x-ray shows diffuse interstitial infiltrates similar to that in PCP. Hypoxemia is invariably present.

Therapy with ganciclovir should be considered when a patient has documented CMV pneumonitis with no other pathogen identified and progressive deterioration.

CNS Infection

Personality changes, difficulty concentrating, headaches, and somnolence with or without fever are frequently present in subacute encephalitis caused by CMV. The diagnosis can only be confirmed by brain biopsy, and isolation of the virus by culture or detection of antigen or nucleic acid. Prompt administration of ganciclovir should be considered in AIDS patients with CMV encephalitis, but no data on its efficacy are yet available. In patients already receiving ganciclovir, it may be reasonable to add or change to foscarnet therapy.

CMV may also cause myelitis or polyradiculopathy, which presents as a spinal cord syndrome with lower limb weakness, spasticity, areflexia, and hypoesthesia. The CSF abnormalities are very unusual for a viral infection (i.e., polymorphonuclear pleocytosis (average cell count 450), increased protein, and moderately low glucose concentration. The disease is progressive, and is fatal in untreated patients. Survival may be increased in patients treated with ganciclovir.

Approach to Treatment

As mentioned earlier, acyclovir is not effective against CMV. Ganciclovir and foscarnet are the two agents currently available with potent anti-CMV activity. Since both agents are Virustatic, chronic suppressive therapy (commonly at a lower dose) is usually required after acute treatment in order to prevent disease progression.

Recent studies in ocular CMV infection have suggested that the two agents are equally efficacious in controlling CMV retinitis (mean time to disease progression 60 to 70 days). There may be a slight improvement in survival for those receiving foscarnet instead of ganciclovir as initial therapy, provided no renal impairment exists. Reasons for this are unclear, and may potentially include increased antiretroviral use with foscarnet (because of nonoverlapping toxicities) and synergistic anti-HIV activity of zidovudine (AZT) and foscarnet (demonstrated in vitro).

However, in most instances, ganciclovir is still preferred as initial therapy because it is easier to administer and is associated with fewer side effects (i.e., greater quality of life) compared to foscarnet. Foscarnet is usually indicated if severe side effects preclude ganciclovir treatment, or when the disease progresses despite treatment with ganciclovir.

On average, IV antiviral therapy is effective at delaying CMV retinitis progression for approximately 60 to 70 days. However, retinitis eventually progresses; this may be due to a number of factors, including the following:

INADEQUATE LOCAL DRUG CONCENTRA-TIONS.   Antiviral concentrations may not be as high in the eye (where the disease is) as in the serum; therefore, progression may occur because of subtherapeutic intraocular drug levels. Potential options to overcome this include the following:

1. *Increase current antiviral dose:* Often, reinstituting therapy at induction doses is effective in halting disease progression; patients who respond may then require continued therapy with higher doses. This may also place these patients at higher risk of experiencing dose-related toxicities.

2. *Administer antiviral locally:* Therapeutic intraocular drug concentrations may be achieved by administering agents

directly in the eye. This may be done by *intravitreal injections*. Experience with intravitreal ganciclovir and limited case reports of intravitreal foscarnet suggest that this route of administration may be effective in controlling disease progression in patients who are failing or are intolerant of systemic antiviral therapy. Intravitreal injections should be done by an experienced ophthalmologist.

If the patient responds to intravitreal ganciclovir injections, one may wish to consider using a *sustained-release intraocular ganciclovir implant*. Once this device is surgically implanted, a constant amount of ganciclovir is released into the eye; the device usually contains enough drug for 6 to 8 months, and thus negates the need for frequent intraocular injections. Although this may certainly be preferable in terms of convenience, implant devices are quite expensive, and may possibly be associated with complications, including increased risk of early retinal detachment.

The implant alone has also been shown to be more effective than IV ganciclovir in delaying progression of CMV retinitis (over 200 days versus 60 to 70 days). However, one should try to continue with systemic ganciclovir therapy if possible, since intraocular administration results in very little systemic drug distribution.

PATIENT INTOLERANCE. As mentioned earlier, ganciclovir and foscarnet are associated with serious toxicities, which may limit the amount of drug one is able to administer. For instance, the main dose-limiting toxicity of ganciclovir is neutropenia, which occurs in up to 40 percent of patients. This not only places patients at risk of infection, but also limits concurrent therapy with other potentially hematosuppressive agents (e.g., zidovudine, TMP-SMX). Potential options to overcome this include the following:

1. *Add another agent to counteract toxicity:* For example, administration of a colony-stimulating factor (e.g., G-CSF) may be effective in counteracting neutropenic effects associated with systemic ganciclovir therapy. However, one must take into consideration the potential side effects associated with this agent, as well as the additional cost and inconvenience.

2. *Switch to an alternative route of administration:* Depending upon the nature or type of drug-related toxicities the patient is experiencing, alternative routes of administration may be considered. At the present time, these alternatives apply only to ganciclovir; foscarnet is only available for IV administration.

(a) Systemic toxicity: If a patient is experiencing considerable toxicity associated with systemic ganciclovir therapy, one may wish to consider *intraocular ganciclovir* administration. Systemic toxicities of ganciclovir may be avoided by administering the agent locally into the eye; in many cases, this route of administration may be even more effective than conventional systemic ganciclovir therapy, since higher amounts of drug are being delivered directly to the site of infection (see No. 1). However, local antiviral therapy is not without its risks; there are many potential immediate and chronic local complications associated with this route of administration.

More importantly, perhaps, are the potential risks associated with lack of systemic drug therapy. CMV is spread hematogenously; thus, although a patient may only be exhibiting signs of infection in the eye, there is the risk that the virus may spread and cause disease in the other eye or even other organs. In a recent trial, two-thirds of CMV retinitis patients who received only local antiviral therapy (with a ganciclovir implant) developed retinitis in the contralateral eye by the end of the study period. The risk of developing CMV disease in other end organs was also increased. Therefore, maintenance systemic therapy should be attempted or encouraged if at all possible.

(b) Line-related complications: If a patient is experiencing frequent complications associated with a permanent central line, a potential option to consider is *oral ganciclovir.* An oral formulation of ganciclovir has recently been licensed in the United States and Canada for CMV retinitis maintenance therapy. Oral administration would avoid the need for installing a permanent IV line, with subsequently less risk of sepsis and line-related events, and added patient convenience. The efficacy of oral ganciclovir as maintenance therapy for CMV retinitis has been demonstrated in a number of recent trials; however, there may be a slight advantage in terms of delaying disease progression (i.e., extra 5 to 12 days) with IV ganciclovir compared to oral. This difference may be due to slightly higher drug concentrations achieved with IV administration compared to oral. The oral formulation should only be used in patients with proper gastrointestinal absorption; other issues such as potential drug interactions and cost need to be considered.

VIRAL DRUG RESISTANCE. With prolonged therapy, viral resistance may develop; this should be suspected especially if a patient does not respond to reinstitution of higher doses of the current agent. Potential management options in this case include the following:

1. *Switch agents:* Ganciclovir resistance often occurs when the infected cells are not able to phosphorylate the drug to its active form; since foscarnet does not need to be phosphorylated, it is often effective against ganciclovir-resistant CMV. Conversely, however, it is unclear whether foscarnet-resistant CMV will respond to ganciclovir.

2. *Combine agents:* In vitro, ganciclovir and foscarnet have synergistic activity against CMV; thus, using a combination of both agents may be effective in a patient who is currently failing monotherapy. The optimal doses for combination therapy have not been clearly defined, and should probably be tailored according to individual patient response or toxicity. Ideally, one may be able to use maintenance doses of each agent (in order to minimize toxicity). However, some patients may require induction doses of one or both agents in order to prevent disease progression. Disadvantages of combination therapy include increased risk of toxicity, decreased convenience (i.e., a patient could potentially spend several hours of a day receiving IV infusions and hydration therapy), and increased cost.

PROGRESSION OF HIV DISEASE.   As HIV infection advances, the patient's condition may continue to deteriorate, and retinitis may eventually progress as well. At all times during the course of disease, the risks and benefits of therapy need to be carefully weighed.

Antiviral Agents

Ganciclovir (Cytovene)

Ganciclovir is a nucleoside analog, which is phosphorylated in CMV-infected cells to its active triphosphate form. The triphosphate acts as a chain terminator, thus inhibiting viral DNA synthesis. Previously, ganciclovir was only available in IV formulation; more recently, new formulations of ganciclovir have been developed, allowing administration either orally or intraocularly via sustained-release implants. Since ganciclovir is excreted by the kidneys, dosage adjustment is necessary in patients with impaired renal function (Table 8–11).

TABLE 8–11

Ganciclovir Dosage Guidelines for Renal Impairment

CREATININE CLEARANCE* (ML/1.73M²/MIN)	IV GANCICLOVIR INDUCTION DOSE (DOUBLE DOSING INTERVAL FOR MAINTENANCE THERAPY)
≥80	5 mg/kg q12h
50–79	2.5 mg/kg q12h
25–49	2.5 mg/kg q24h
<25	1.25 mg/kg q24h
CreatinineClearance (mL/min)	**Oral Ganciclovir Dose**
≥70	1000 mg TID
50–69	1500 mg daily or 500 mg TID
25–49	1000 mg daily or 500 mg TID
10–24	500 mg daily
<10	500 mg 3x/week, after dialysis

*Creatinine clearance (CrCl) can be calculated by the following formulas:

$$CrCl\ (mL/min) = \frac{(140 - age,\ years)\ (Ideal\ body\ weight,\ kg)}{50 \times (serum\ creatinine,\ \mu mol/L)} \times 60$$

$$CrCl\ (mL/1.73m^2/min) = \frac{(140 - age,\ years)\ (Ideal\ body\ weight,\ kg)}{50 \times (serum\ creatinine,\ \mu mol/L)} \times 60 \times \frac{1.73}{(BSA,\ m^2)}$$

CrCl for females = 0.85 × above value

IV ADMINISTRATION.   Induction: 5 mg/kg IV (infuse at constant rate over 1 hour) q12h for 14 to 21 days (or until retinitis is stabilized).

Maintenance: 5 mg/kg IV once daily, or 6 mg/kg IV once daily 5 days/week.

Toxicity frequently limits therapy with ganciclovir. The main side effects are hematologic. *Neutropenia* (absolute neutrophil count [ANC] <1000/mm³) occurs in 40 percent of ganciclovir recipients. It usually occurs early (i.e., induction period or early maintenance), but may occur later in therapy as well. It is usually reversible, but irreversible neutropenia has been reported. Concurrent administration of other hematotoxic agents should be done with caution. The dosage should be reduced when ANC<1000/mm³ or discontinued when severe neutropenia occurs (ANC<500/mm³). Use of a colony-stimulating factor (e.g., G-CSF) may be effective in counteracting neutropenia, and thus allow continued administration of ganciclovir.

Thrombocytopenia (platelet count <20,000/mm^3) occurs in 29 percent of AIDS patients receiving the drug.

Other side effects include confusion, dizziness, headache, unusual thoughts, or convulsions. Gastrointestinal disturbances, with nausea, vomiting, abnormal liver function tests, and diarrhea, are not uncommon. (Appendix 1 presents further details and comments on management.) Approximately one-third of patients must discontinue or interrupt IV ganciclovir treatment.

ORAL ADMINISTRATION.   The oral bioavailability of ganciclovir is quite low (6 to 9 percent). Therefore, the dosages required are considerably higher than those conventionally used for IV therapy. Bioavailability is increased approximately 20 percent when the drug is taken with food. The recommended dose for CMV retinitis maintenance therapy is 1 g PO TID with food; as with intravenous administration, dosage should be adjusted for renal function (Table 8–11).

In comparison to IV administration, oral ganciclovir is associated with reduced risk of sepsis and catheter events. The incidence of gastrointestinal events (e.g., diarrhea, nausea, anorexia, vomiting) is approximately equal. There may be a decreased risk of neutropenia and anemia with oral ganciclovir; this may be due to slightly lower serum drug concentrations after oral versus IV administration.

Use of the oral formulation should be avoided in patients with concurrent gastrointestinal conditions (e.g., opportunistic infections, enteropathy, diarrhea), which may limit drug absorption. Other considerations include potential drug interactions (i.e., [ddI] didanosine, see Appendix 3) and cost (approximately $39 US/day). The role of oral ganciclovir in the prophylaxis of CMV retinitis is controversial; the potential risk of inducing ganciclovir-resistant CMV strains is of concern, since current options for management are limited. Thus, the routine use of oral ganciclovir for this indication is currently not approved.

INTRAVITREAL INJECTIONS.   Intravitreal ganciclovir injections should be done by an experienced ophthalmologist. Usually, it is recommended that the dose be injected 3 to 4 mm from the corneoscleral limbus in the inferotemporal quadrant using a tuberculin syringe and a 30-gauge needle under topical anesthesia.

Dosing protocols may vary from institution to institution. Usually, doses of 200 to 400 μg ganciclovir are injected intravitreally every 2 to 3 days as induction therapy, and then once a week as maintenance therapy.

Immediate side effects include transient increase in intraocular pressure, temporary ocular pain, and total amaurosis for up to 10 minutes postinjection. Potential long-term complications include ocular infection, lens damage, subconjunctival hemorrhage, retinal detachment, and optic nerve atrophy.

If at all possible, concurrent systemic antiviral therapy should be considered in order to decrease the risk of developing CMV disease in the contralateral eye or other end-organs.

INTRAOCULAR IMPLANTS.   If prolonged local administration of ganciclovir is desirable, sustained-release intraocular ganciclovir implants may be a potential therapeutic option. These devices release a constant amount of ganciclovir into the eye for a period of 6 to 8 months, and thus are considerably more convenient than frequent intravitreal injections.

These implants are available from Chiron Vision (for more information, call 1-800-263-3557 [Canada] or 1-800-553-3354 [United States]), and cost approximately $5000 each. Thus, one may wish to start with a short trial of intravitreal injections (in order to confirm that the patient will respond to higher ocular antiviral concentrations) before committing to surgical implantation of an expensive ocular implant.

Potential disadvantages include risks associated with the surgical procedure, ocular infection, and retinal detachment. As stated with intravitreal injections, concurrent systemic antiviral therapy should be considered in order to decrease the risk of developing CMV disease in the contralateral eye or other end organs.

Foscarnet (Foscavir)

Foscarnet is a pyrophosphate that inhibits the DNA polymerase of CMV by blocking the pyrophosphate-binding site of the enzyme and preventing cleavage. It does not require intracellular phosphorylation, and therefore may be effective against ganciclovir-resistant strains of CMV that lack the phosphorylating enzymes required to convert ganciclovir to its active form.

The standard foscarnet regimen for induction therapy is 60 mg/kg IV q8h, while maintenance regiments of 90 to 120 mg/kg IV once daily are most commonly used. Foscarnet dose should be adjusted regularly based on weight and monitoring of renal status as assessed by estimated creatinine clearance (Table 8–12).

TABLE 8–12

Foscarnet Dosage Guidelines for Renal Impairment

CREATININE CLEARANCE (ML/MIN/KG)	FOSCARNET DOSE (MG/KG)
Induction	
≥1.6	60.0
1.5	56.5
1.4	53.0
1.3	49.4
1.2	45.9
1.1	42.4
1.0	38.9
0.9	35.3
0.8	31.8
0.7	28.3
0.6	24.8
0.5	21.2
0.4	17.7
Maintenance	
≥1.4	90
1.2–1.4	78
1.0–1.2	75
0.8–1.0	71
0.6–0.8	63
0.4–0.8	57

Foscarnet should be infused over 2 hours via an infusion pump (rapid infusion may cause sudden chelation of serum electrolytes, including calcium, potentially leading to arrythmias). Adequate hydration with 500 to 1000 ml normal saline prior to infusion is necessary to minimize renal impairment.

Commonly occurring side effects include mild headache, fatigue, nausea, and fever. Renal impairment can occur in up to one-third of patients receiving foscarnet; thus, frequent measurement of renal function is recommended, and dose adjustments should be made as necessary. Other side effects include electrolyte abnormalities (e.g., hypokalemia, hypocalcemia, hypomagnesemia), neutropenia, anemia, increased liver function tests, and seizures. Penile ulcers have also been observed with drug administration (see Appendix 1 for further details and comments on management).

Indications for Admission

- All patients starting treatment with ganciclovir or foscarnet need admission, or administration of the first dose under observation in a medical day unit.

- Patients changing from one drug to another need admission or observation in medical day units.

- Arrangements should be made for central line placement on admission or prior to drug administration in a medical day unit. Patient education on drug self-administration, and home care arrangements should be done in either setting.

Follow-up

- Patients should be seen weekly for 1 to 2 months to monitor hematology and blood chemistries and re-evaluate drug dose.

- If stable, follow-up can be extended to every 2 weeks.

- Ophthalmologic assessment for patients with CMV retinitis should be done every 4 to 8 weeks.

Suggested Readings

Ward-Able C, Phillips P, Tsoukas CM. The use of oral ganciclovir in the treatment of cytomegalovirus retinitis in patients with AIDS. Can Med Assoc J 1996;154:363–8.

Jacobson MA. Current management of cytomegalovirus disease in patients with AIDS. AIDS Res Hum Retr 1994;10:917–23.

Polis MA, Masur H. Promising new treatments for cytomegalovirus retinitis. JAMA 1995;273:1457–9.

HERPES SIMPLEX VIRUS

Tong Yeung, M.D., B.B.S., M.R.C.P.(U.K.), F.C.C.P.

Mary Fanning, M.D., Ph.D., F.R.C.P.C., F.A.C.P.

Primary herpes simplex virus (HSV) infection is followed by viral latency in the nerve root ganglia corresponding to the initial infection site. Latent HSV often reactivates in immunosuppressed people and can cause severe recurrent disease with extensive tissue destruction and prolonged viral shedding. Ulcerative HSV infection lasting longer than 1 month is diagnostic of AIDS.

The incubation period of primary HSV infection ranges from 2 to 12 days. The frequency and severity of recurrent HSV infection increases with increasing immunosuppression, symptoms possibly persisting for several weeks.

Common HSV infection sites are orolabial, genital, and anorectal. Occasionally esophagitis and encephalitis may occur. In adults with AIDS, HSV encephalitis usually arises as a complication of primary or reactivated orolabial HSV infection. Diagnosis is difficult and may require a brain biopsy.

Diagnosis can usually be made clinically. The Tzanck smear is prepared with cells from the base of a fresh vesicular lesion, stained with Wright or Giemsa stain and examined for typical, multinucleate giant cells. It takes only hours to get a result but does not distinguish herpes zoster from simplex. Cells from the base of a fresh vesicular lesion must be collected for direct immunofluorescent techniques, which also give a rapid diagnosis within hours and are more sensitive and specific for either simplex or zoster. Vesicular fluid collected in a tuberculine syringe should be submitted for culture—still the gold standard for HSV diagnosis, usually taking 3-4 days. It is the only test suitable for the diagnosis of asymptomatic shedding, as well as for antiviral susceptibility.

Acyclovir is the antiviral agent of choice for most HSV infections among AIDS patients. The route of administration, dosage, and duration of therapy depend on the site and severity of the acute HSV infection—it has slightly higher activity against HSV-1 than HSV-2. Acyclovir permeates all tissues, including the brain and CSF, and is cleared by renal mechanism.

Dosage Adjustment of IV Acyclovir in Patients with Renal Dysfunction

Table 8–13 presents dosage adjustment recommendations based on creatinine clearance.

TABLE 8–13

Dosage Adjustment of Acyclovir in Renal Dysfunction

CREATININE CLEARANCE (ML/MIN/1.73M^2)	% OF STANDARD DOSE*	DOSAGE INTERVAL (HR)
>50	100	8
25–50	100	12
10–25	100	24
0–10	50	24

*Usually 5 mg/kg; 10 mg/kg for HSV infection involving visceral organs and varicella-zoster virus infection.

Management

Mucocutaneous Infection, Mild	Acyclovir 200 mg 5 times/day (PO)
Mucocutaneous Infection, Severe	Acyclovir 15 mg/kg/day (IV) in three divided doses
Visceral Organ Infection	Acyclovir 30 mg/kg/day IV
Recurrent Mucocutaneous Infection	Acyclovir 200 to 400 mg TID or QID.
Severe Infection Caused by Acyclovir-Resistant HSV	Foscarnet 40 mg/kg IV TID or acyclovir 1.5 to 2.0 mg/kg/hr continuous infusion.

Treatment with acyclovir should continue until all mucocutaneous lesions have crusted or reepithelialized. The duration of treatment is usually 7 to 14 days. For life-threatening HSV infection or visceral organ involvement, treatment should last at least 10 days, but longer therapy may be necessary. If the lesion does not heal, repeat viral cultures should be obtained, high-dose IV therapy (30 mg/kg/day) should be given, and acyclovir-resistant HSV infection should be ruled out.

Most acyclovir-resistant strains isolated from AIDS patients have been thymidine kinase-deficient, and have remained susceptible in vitro to vidarabine, which is phosphorylated without thymidine kinase and foscarnet, and does not require phosphorylation for activity. A recent comparative trial shows that foscarnet is superior to vidarabine for treating acyclovir-resistant HSV and is far less toxic. Chronic prophylaxis with daily acyclovir 200 to 400 mg PO TID, or foscarnet 40 mg/kg/day IV should be considered in patients successfully treated for acyclovir-resistant HSV.

VARICELLA-ZOSTER VIRUS

Tong Yeung, M.D., B.B.S., M.R.C.P.(U.K.), F.C.C.P.

Mary Fanning, M.D., Ph.D., F.R.C.P.C., F.A.C.P.

Primary Infection—Varicella

In healthy, immunocompetent children varicella is usually a benign illness. Adults, however, are more likely to develop complications during primary varicella-zoster virus (VZV) infection and infection spreads to visceral organs (e.g., lung, liver) in up to one-third of immunocompetent adults with primary infection. Although most adults with AIDS have been previously infected with VZV and are not susceptible to primary infection, for those who are, a protracted and potentially life-threatening illness could ensue.

Recurrent Zoster Infection

The illness usually begins with radicular pain, followed by a localized, erythematous rash covering one to three dermatomes. The patient experiences increasing pain and the maculopapules progress to fluid-filled vesicles. Occasionally, widespread cutaneous or visceral dissemination may occur. Involvement of the lung, liver, or CNS may be life threatening.

Management

Primary Infection	Acyclovir 30 mg/kg/day IV or 600 to 800 mg 5 times/day PO.
Recurrent Infection, Localized Zoster	Acyclovir 30 mg/kg/day IV or 600 to 800 mg 5 times/day PO.
Recurrent Infection, Disseminated	Acyclovir 30 mg/kg/day IV.
Severe Infection Caused by Acyclovir-Resistant VZV	Foscarnet 40 mg/kg BID IV.

Immunocompromised people with primary or recurrent VZV infection treated with IV acyclovir exhibit less viral shedding, reduced formation of new lesions, less chance of dissemination, and lower mortality rates. Treatment should be continued for at least 7 days or until all external lesions are crusted.

References

HERPES SIMPLEX VIRUS

1. Sande MA, Volberding PA. The Medical Management of AIDS. 4th ed., Philadelphia: WB Saunders, 1994.

Suggested Reading

VARICELLA-ZOSTER VIRUS

Sande MA, Volberding PA. The Medical Management of AIDS. 4th ed. Philadelphia: WB Saunders, 1994.

■ HISTOPLASMOSIS

Mary Fanning, M.D., Ph.D., F.R.C.P.C., F.A.C.P.

Histoplasmosis often affects HIV-positive individuals who have lived in or travelled to endemic areas such as the Caribbean, Central and South America, major river valleys in the United States and Canada (such as the Ohio–Mississippi River valley and the St. Lawrence River valley). But evidence of exposure may be elusive since it usually represents reactivation of an original infection owing to severe immune deficiency.

Presenting symptoms are nonspecific and include persistent fever and weight loss, perhaps also oropharyngeal ulcers, intestinal ulceration, skin lesions, hepatosplenomegaly, pancytopenia, and interstitial pneumonia.

Diagnosis is with special stains (periodic acid–Schiff and silver stains) and culture of bone marrow and other affected tissues. Occasionally, blood smear or blood cultures will yield the organism.

The treatment of choice is amphotericin B 0.5 to 0.6 mg/kg IV daily to a total dose of 2 g, or at least 4 to 8 weeks, or itraconazole 200 mg PO BID, followed by life-long suppressive therapy: itraconazole 200 mg PO BID or amphotericin B 0.5 to 0.8 mg/kg IV weekly or biweekly. Ketoconazole may be used as suppressive therapy, but relapse is more common (60 percent) than with amphotericin B (10 to 20 percent).

Suggested Readings

Drugs for AIDS and associated infections. *Med Lett* 1995;37:87–94.
Sarosi GA, Johnson PC. Disseminated histoplasmosis in patients infected with human immunodeficiency virus. Clin Infect Dis 1992;14 (Suppl 1): 560–67.

■ MYCOBACTERIUM AVIUM COMPLEX INFECTION

Ahmed Bayoumi, M.D., F.R.C.P.C.

Microbiology

Mycobacterium avium complex (MAC), previously named *Mycobacterium avium*-intracellulare (MAI), is a group of closely related serovars of two species, *M. avium* and *M. intracellulare.* In patients with AIDS, 97 percent of isolates are *M. avium.*

Epidemiology

The incidence of MAC is increasing as patients survive longer and surveillance techniques improve. In the era of PCP prophylaxis, 30 to 40 percent of AIDS patients will, at some point, develop MAC, and 13 percent of them will have MAC as their first AIDS-defining illness. The most important risk factor for the development of MAC is a low CD4 count, with the risk being low at a CD4 count >75, but increasing exponentially as the CD4 count drops further. In one study, the median CD4 count at the time of diagnosis was 11. The presence of another AIDS-defining illness, particularly CMV disease, also increases the risk of developing MAC. Gender, racial or ethnic group, and mode of acquisition of HIV are not risk factors for the development of MAC.

Pathogenesis

MAC is almost always the result of a primary infection, rather than reactivation. MAC has been isolated in the drinking water supply of many large cities as well as in soil, plants, bedding, house dust, and dairy products. Recent reports have suggested that hospital water supplies may be an important source.

Colonization of the gastrointestinal tract or, less commonly, the respiratory tract may precede dissemination by 4 to 5 months, but does not do so in every case.

Clinical Manifestations

Disseminated MAC is commoner than localized infection. At presentation, patients usually have a 2- to 6-week history of signs and symptoms, with the most common being fever, night sweats, weight loss, fatigue, diarrhea, lymphadenopathy, abdominal pain, and hepatosplenomegaly. Almost any organ can be involved with localized infection, although this is rare. An elevated alkaline phosphatase and anemia are both very common laboratory abnormalities. Anemia has been identified as an independent predictor of a poor prognosis.

The median survival after a diagnosis of MAC has been consistently described as between 107 and 139 days, although with treatment, patients may live up to twice as long. MAC is unlikely to be the immediate cause of death but contributes to mortality through wasting and organ dysfunction.

Diagnosis

The clinical diagnosis of MAC can be difficult, as the findings are relatively nonspecific in late-stage HIV disease. Blood cultures are positive 86 to 98 percent of the time. Susceptibility testing generally does not predict sensitivity of MAC to antibiotics, although a recent study of clarithromycin sensitivity using the radiometric technique did show a correlation. This has not been shown for other antibiotics.

Prophylaxis

Rifabutin has been recommended for prophylaxis of MAC in patients with a CD4 count of <75, although some clinicians will wait until the CD4 count is <50. The original recommendation was to initiate prophylaxis at a CD4 count of 100. Active tuberculosis should be ruled out before the initiation of prophylaxis. Evidence from clinical trials shows that patients not receiving rifabutin are 2.2 times more likely to develop MAC than patients receiving the drug. Despite this, rifabutin has been only partially adopted into therapy because of concerns such as the development of resistance, side effects, drug interactions, polypharmacy, and cost.

Clarithromycin has also been reported to be an effective prophylactic agent, although the results have not been published and formally reviewed at the time of publication of this manuscript. Trials of combination therapy for prophylaxis are continuing.

Treatment

A U.S. Public Health Services Task Force has recommended that MAC be treated with a minimum of two drugs, one of which is a macrolide (clarithromycin or azithromycin), although many clinicians would start with at least three. Most clinicians would include ethambutol in a treatment regimen. Preliminary results of the Canadian randomized open-label trial for combination therapy for MAC bacteremia showed that there was a benefit in mortality and morbidity when *clarithromycin, ethambutol, and rifabutin* are used in combination (compared to another protocol), suggesting that this is a reasonable initial therapy for patients with MAC. The treatment of MAC must be individualized to

TABLE 8–14

Drug Therapy for MAC

CLASS	DRUG	DOSE
Macrolides	Clarithromycin	500–1000 mg PO BID
	Azithromycin	600 mg PO daily
Quinolones	Ciprofloxacin	500–750 mg PO BID
	Ofloxacin	400 mg PO BID
Rifamycins	Rifabutin	300–600 mg PO daily
	Rifampin	10 mg/kg/day PO (max 600 mg)
Aminoglycosides	Amikacin	7.5–15 mg/kg/day IV
Other	Ethambutol	15–25 mg/kg/day PO
	Clofazimine	100 mg PO daily

provide the patient with the best symptom control and the least drug toxicity. Treatment is continued for life. Isoniazid and pyrazinamide are *not* effective against MAC. Current drugs available for the treatment of MAC are given in Table 8–14.

Suggested Readings

Benson C. Disseminated *Mycobacterium avium* complex disease in patients with AIDS. AIDS Res Human Retrovir 1994;10:913–6.

Benson CA. Treatment of disseminated disease due to the *Mycobacterium avium* complex in patients with AIDS. Clin Infect Dis 1994;18(Suppl 3):S237–42.

Gordin F, Masur H. Prophylaxis of *Mycobacterium avium* complex bacteremia in patients with AIDS. Clin Infect Dis 1994;18(Suppl 3):S223–6.

Inderlied CB, Kemper CA, Bermudez LEM. The *Mycobacterium avium* complex. Clin Microbiol Rev 1993;6:266–310.

PNEUMOCYSTIS CARINII PNEUMONIA

Charles Chan, M.D., F.R.C.P.C., F.C.C.P., F.A.C.P.

Despite major advances in the prophylaxis of *Pneumocystis carinii* pneumonia (PCP) during the past decade, PCP is still the most common opportunistic infection in patients with HIV infection. Up to 85 percent of HIV-infected patients will develop PCP at some time during the course of their disease, and experience significant morbidity and mortality as a consequence. Failure of initial therapy, requiring a switch to another agent, can occur in 6 to 10 percent with mild PCP. For those with severe PCP (initial PO_2 <70 mmHg and $(A–a)O_2D$>35), failure of therapy may be as frequent as 19 to 82 percent. This is reduced by two- to threefold when adjunctive corticosteroids are given. Mortality rates are 2 to 6 percent for mild cases and 10 to 92 percent for moderate to severe cases. Respiratory failure requiring ventilation is associated with mortality as high as 50 percent. The prognosis in these cases is better if respiratory failure occurs in the first few days of therapy and the patient's baseline performance status was good prior to PCP. Long-term sequelae include formation of pulmonary bullae or blebs, fibrotic changes, and recurrent pneumothoraces during and after therapy. These changes lead to reduced pulmonary reserve and reduced exercise tolerance. Survival for patients in whom PCP is the AIDS-defining illness is approximately 50 percent at 24 months and 36 percent at 36 months.

Presenting symptoms include a dry, nonproductive cough, insidious onset of shortness of breath, fever, weight loss, malaise, and fatigue. Patients on suboptimal PCP prophylaxis may have a somewhat longer course of illness and less impressive chest x-ray changes. Furthermore, focal infiltrates on chest x-ray favoring the upper lung zones and perihilar regions are quite common early changes in patients with suboptimal PCP prophylaxis.

Investigations include chest x-ray, arterial blood gases, sputum for PCP, culture and sensitivity, AFB and mycobacterial culture, pulmonary function tests, and gallium scan (if symptoms are mild), and bronchoscopy with bronchoalveolar lavage if other investigations are negative. The bronchoscopy may be done after therapy has been initiated and is useful even after 5 to 7 days of effective treatment.

Concurrent bacterial infections (*Streptococcus, Haemophilus, Staphylococcus,* and *Pseudomonas*) are becoming more frequent. Suspect a concurrent bacterial process if the WBC is high (7 to 10 range) and blood pressure is low, with or without consolidation/cavitation on the chest x-ray.

Treatment

Criteria for admission include the following:

- PO_2 <70 mmHg.
- Unable to take oral therapy.

- Compliance expected to be poor.
- Appears toxic or severely compromised.

IV Therapy

IV is begun in the following circumstances:

- Patient is acutely ill.
- Patient is unable to take oral therapy.
- PO_2 <70 mmHg.

TRIMETHOPRIM-SULFAMETHOXAZOLE. Trimethoprim (20 mg/kg/day)–sulfamethoxazole (TMP-SMX) IV q6h for 21 days (may be adjusted to TMP 15 mg/kg/day after clinical improvement at about 1 week).

PENTAMIDINE. Pentamidine 4 mg/kg/day IV over 1 to 3 hours then 3 mg/kg/day at about 1 week to complete 14 to 21 days.

CLINDAMYCIN-PRIMAQUINE. Clindamycin 600 mg q8h plus primaquine 15 to 30 mg PO daily for 14 to 21 days.

TRIMETREXATE. Trimetrexate 45 mg/M^2 daily IV plus leucovorin 20 mg/M^2 q6h IV/PO for 21 days.

ADJUVANT THERAPY. Corticosteroids can be added if PO_2 <70 mmHg or $(A–a)O_2D$ gradient >40 mmHg. As the clinical course is usually unstable in the first 3 to 5 days of treatment, corticosteroids can stabilize the clinical situation and may avoid hypoxemic respiratory failure and the need of positive-pressure ventilatory support.

Prednisone 40 mg PO BID for 7 days, then 40 mg daily for 7 days, then 20 mg daily for 7 days.

Switch from IV to oral regimen when patient improves. Change therapy if patient worsens after 4 days or is not improved after 7 to 10 days.

Oral Therapy

TMP-SMX. TMP-SMX 2 DS tablets PO TID to QID for 21 days.

DAPSONE-TMP. Dapsone 100 mg PO/day plus TMP 200 mg PO QID (15 mg/kg/day) for 21 days.

ATOVAQUONE. Atovaquone oral suspension 1500 mg PO daily or tablet formulation 750 mg PO TID with food for 21 days.

CLINDAMYCIN-PRIMAQUINE. Clindamycin 300 to 450 mg PO QID plus primaquine 15 mg base PO/day for 21 days.

Side Effects

TMP-SMX.   Rash, fever, leukopenia, hepatitis, thrombocytopenia at 1 to 2 weeks.

PENTAMIDINE.   Hypotension, renal failure, elevated liver function enzymes, hypoglycemia, hyperglycemia, pancreatitis, arrhythmias.

ATOVAQUONE.   Rash, fever, diarrhea.

CLINDAMYCIN-PRIMAQUINE.   Rash, gastrointestinal side effects, *clostridium difficile* colitis methemoglobinemia.

TRIMETREXATE.   Anemia, leukopenia, thrombocytopenia, fever, rash.

Prophylaxis

After completing therapy everyone should be initiated on long-term prophylaxis. Other indications are CD4 count <200 (15 percent), a history of prior PCP, recurrent thrush, or unexplained fevers.

Possible prophylaxis regimens include the following:

- TMP-SMX 1 DS tablet daily or three times weekly.

- Dapsone 100 mg daily (or 2 to 3 times/week) plus TMP 200 mg/day.

- Aerosol pentamidine 300 mg q 2 to 4 weeks via Respigard nebulizer.

- Pentamidine 4 mg/kg IV q 2 to 4 weeks.

- Atovaquone suspension 1500 mg/day or tablet 750 mg TID.

Suggested Readings

Carr A, Tidall B, Brew BJ, et al. Low-dose trimethoprim-sulfamethoxazole prophylaxis for toxoplasmic encephalitis in patients with AIDS. Ann Intern Med 1992; 177:106–11.

Girard PM, Landman R, Gaudebout C, et al. Dapsone/pyrimethamine compared with aerosolized pentamidine as primary prophylaxis against *Pneumocystis carinii* pneumonia and toxoplasmosis in HIV infection. N Engl J Med 1993; 328:1514–20.

Hardy WD, Feinberg J, Finkelstein DM, et al. A controlled trial of trimethoprim-sulfamethoxazole or aerosolized pentamidine for secondary prophylaxis of *Pneumocystis carinii* pneumonia in patients with acquired immunodeficiency syndrome. N Engl J Med 1992;327:1842–8.

Nightengale SD, Carmeron DW, Gordin FM, et al. Two controlled trials of rifabutin prophylaxis against *Mycobacterium avium* complex infection in AIDS. N Engl J Med 1993: 329:828–33.

Recommendations for prophylaxis against *Pneumocystis carinii* pneumonia for adults and adolescents infected with human immunodeficiency virus. MMWR 1992; 41:1–10.

Schneider MME, Hopelman AIM, Schattenkerk JKME, et al. A controlled trial of aerosolized pentamidine or trimethoprim-sulfamethoxazole as a primary prophylaxis against *Pneumocystis carinii pneumonia* in patients with acquired immunodeficiency syndrome. N Engl J Med 1992; 327:1836–41.

TOXOPLASMOSIS

Krystyna Ostrowska, M.D., F.R.C.P.C.

Toxoplasmosis in HIV-positive patients almost always represents a reactivation of latent infection from tissue cysts of *Toxoplasma gondi.* Primary toxoplasmosis, with undetectable levels of IgG antibodies, accounts for less than 5 percent of cases. Approximately 30 percent of AIDS patients develop toxoplasmic encephalitis, which is the most common reason for multifocal brain lesions. Toxoplasmosis is unlikely in patients with CD4 counts >200.

Patients present with subacute (days to weeks) onset of any of the following: headache, fevers, hemiparesis, aphasia, ataxia, seizures, and confusion.

The brain CT scan typically shows rounded, single or multiple, ring-enhancing lesions in cerebral cortex or basal ganglia. The MRI may demonstrate multiple lesions that appear single on CT scans. Single, nonenhancing lesions do not exclude the diagnosis. None of the CT findings are pathognomonic. Definitive diagnosis can only be obtained by brain biopsy, which should be considered if empiric treatment fails to produce clinical or radiologic improvement after 10 to 14 days or if toxoplasmic serology is negative. At the completion of induction therapy, patients should receive life-long maintenance therapy, since the toxoplasma cysts are impermeable by currently available therapeutics.

Indications for Admission

- Decreased level of consciousness (encephalitic form).
- Grand mal seizures or status epilepticus.
- Evidence of increased intracranial pressure (clinically and on CT).
- Severe neurologic impairment with inability to cope at home.
- Severe side effects and intolerance of therapy (rash with systemic symptoms, severe diarrhea).

Treatment

Primary Therapy: 6 weeks

Pyrimethamine (Daraprim) plus	200 mg loading dose, then 50 to 75 mg/day PO (max 100 mg/day)
Folinic Acid (leucovorin) plus	25 mg/day PO
Sulfadiazine	4 to 8 g/day PO

If the patient is allergic to sulfa drugs, treatment should be

Clindamycin plus	900 to 1200 mg IV q6–8h or 600 mg q6h PO
Pyrimethamine/ Folinic Acid	(see dosage above)

Chronic Maintenance

Pyrimethamine plus	25 to 50 mg/day PO
Folinic acid (leucovorin) plus	25 mg/day PO
Sulfadiazine	2 g/day PO

If the patient is allergic to sulfa drugs, therapy should be

Clindamycin plus	300 to 450 mg PO q6–8h PO
Pyrimethamine/ Folinic Acid	(see dosage above)

Follow-Up

For induction treatment:

- Once a week for 2 weeks.
- At the end of second week, repeat CT scan.
- Decision regarding continuation of therapy (if responding to treatment) or brain biopsy.
- If responding, visits every 2 weeks.
- At 6 weeks change to maintenance therapy and visits every 1 to 2 months

Suggested Readings

(See Suggested Readings for CNS Manifestations.)

Dannemann BR. Toxoplasmic encephalitis in AIDS. Hosp Pract March 1989; 139–54.

Leift BY, Remington JS. Toxoplasmic encephalitis. Clin Infect Dis 1992, 15:211–22.

TUBERCULOSIS

Mary Fanning, M.D., Ph.D., F.R.C.P.C., F.A.C.P.
Susan Shurtleff, R.N., C.I.C.

Tuberculosis (TB) has resurfaced alongside HIV infection, primarily because of the immunologic defect caused by HIV, that is, progressive depletion of CD4 cells and monocyte/macrophage function defects. Consequently, individuals with both TB and HIV infection have a very high rate of TB reactivation (80 percent/year) compared with the lifetime reactivation rate of 10 percent seen in non-HIV-infected people. In addition, transmission rates are very high in those with HIV (up to 45 percent) and new TB infection can be as prevalent as reactivation. Multi-drug-resistant TB has also appeared among AIDS patients. To date, the incidence of tuberculosis in Canadian HIV populations is low, but vigilance is essential.

TB can precede an AIDS-defining illness in 60 percent of patients and may arise at CD4 counts as high as 400. The disease profile differs in early from advanced HIV disease. However, extrapulmonary infection is common in both groups, occurring in more than 70 percent of those diagnosed with AIDS and in 25 to 45 percent before AIDS diagnosis is confirmed. The most frequent manifestations of TB include lymphadenitis, bacteremia, and CNS-tuberculous abscesses and tuberculomas. Blood cultures may be positive in up to 40 percent. TB skin tests are positive more frequently early in HIV infection (71 percent) than in those with more advanced disease (33 percent).

Pulmonary infection is frequent, occurring in 74 to 100 percent of patients, and should always be looked for as this is the primary transmission route. However, the physical findings and symptoms of TB are hard to distinguish from those other HIV-associated pulmonary conditions. A chest x-ray and sputum examination for AFB are essential. In patients with relatively preserved immune function and positive TB skin tests, chest x-ray findings are similar to those of reactivation TB in immunocompetent patients, and include cavitation and upper-lobe infiltrates. As immune suppression progresses, the findings become more typical of primary tuberculosis in immunocompetent patients: hilar adenopathy, pleural effusions, and a miliary pattern.

Diagnosis depends on isolation of mycobacteria from sputum, bronchoalveolar lavage, and aspirate of other infected tissues, including blood, CSF, and lymph node aspirate or biopsy. A head CT scan is necessary to diagnose CNS infection, should CNS symptoms be present. An adequate number of sputum samples must be collected to ensure prompt diagnosis. Mycobacterial TB must be differentiated from atypical mycobacteria, such as MAI/MAC, which causes disease in HIV-infected individuals. A delay in diagnosis can lead to increased mortality and TB transmission.

Multi-drug-resistant TB has emerged as a real problem in this population, in whom primary cases develop from exposure to others infected with multi-drug-resistant TB. Secondary cases emerge as a result of poor compliance with therapy and incomplete treatment.

Treatment

Isoniazid (INH) 300 mg/day, rifampin 600 mg/day, and pyrazinamide 25 mg/kg/day for 2 months, followed by INH and rifampin for 7 months or 6 months after culture is negative, whichever is longer.

If INH drug resistance is suspected start INH 300 mg/day, rifampin 600 mg/day, pyrazinamide 25 mg/kg/day, and ethambutol 15 mg/kg/day. Once INH resistance is confirmed, treat with rifampin, ethambutol, and pyrazinamide for 2 months, followed by rifampin and ethambutol for 18 months or 12 months after cultures are negative, whichever is longer.

If rifampin intolerance occurs treat with INH, pyrazinamide, and ethambutol for 18 months to 24 months or for 12 months after culture is negative, whichever is longer.

If multi-drug resistance occurs, treat with at least three drugs to which the isolate is sensitive. Alternative drugs include streptomycin, cycloserine, ethionamide, PAS, ciprofloxacin, and clofazimine, among others.

While treating people with TB it is equally important to prevent the spread of the disease, particularly among other highly susceptible HIV-infected individuals. Hence, infection control guidelines should be strictly followed.

Infection Control Guidelines for the HIV Patient Admitted for Investigation

- In the Emergency Department any patient with HIV infection and a cough should be put in a single room on respiratory precautions.

- Any HIV patient admitted with an undiagnosed cough should be put in a single room on respiratory precautions.

- Three sputum specimens for AFB stain and mycobacterial culture should be ordered (one per day) and collected starting on the day of admission.

- If the first specimen is negative for AFB and an alternative diagnosis is established, microbiologically, discontinue respiratory precautions *but* continue to collect two additional sputum specimens for AFB stain.

- If no alternative diagnosis is established *and* if three consecutive sputum specimens or a BAL is smear negative for AFB, discontinue respiratory precautions.

- If three sputum specimens are not collected within 48 hours, and the patient *is not* responding to medical therapy, a bronchoscopy should be done and a sample sent for AFB smear and mycobacterial culture.

- If three sputum specimens are not collected within 48 hours and the patient is responding to medical therapy after 72 hours, discontinue respiratory precautions.

- If the sputum is positive for AFB, continue respiratory precautions during treatment and discharge as soon as the patient's medical condition allows.

- If a patient known to have MOTT (mycobacteria other than *Mycobacterium* TB) presents with nonpulmonary symptoms and the respiratory symptomatology is unchanged, respiratory precautions are not required.

- If a patient known to have MOTT presents with worsening respiratory symptoms, treat as an undiagnosed cough, as outlined above.

Infection Control Guidelines for a Patient Undergoing Treatment for Tuberculosis

- If the patient remains hospitalized with a diagnosis of *Mycobacterium* TB, continue respiratory precautions for 12 weeks and obtain three negative sputum specimens for AFB smear prior to discontinuation of respiratory precautions.

- If a patient with a diagnosis of *Mycobacterium* TB is discharged home, recommend the use of a high-particulate-filter mask if the person is in contact with other people for 5 minutes or more.

- If the patient with a diagnosis of *Mycobacterium* TB needs to be seen in a health care facility, such as a clinic, medical day care unit, doctor's office, or pharmacy, recommend that the patient wear a high-particulate-filter mask.

Suggested Readings

Barnes PF, Bloch AB, Davidson PT, Snider DE. Tuberculosis in patients with human immunodeficiency virus infection. N Engl J Med 1991; 324:1644–50.

Essential components of a tuberculosis prevention and control program. Screening for tuberculosis and tuberculosis infection in high risk populations. MMWR 1995; 44:(RR-11):1–34.

Nosocomial transmission of multi-drug resistant tuberculosis among HIV-infected persons—Florida and New York, 1988–1991. MMWR 1991; 40:585–91.

US Department of Health and Human Services. Guidelines for Preventing the Transmission of Mycobacterium tuberculosis in Health-Care Facilities, 1994, MMWR 1994; 43, (RR-13): 1–132.

ADVERSE DRUG REACTIONS IN HIV PATIENTS

Alice Tseng, Pharm.D.

Michelle Foisy, Pharm.D.

INCIDENCE

HIV patients often require multiple agents, especially in later stages of illness. Polypharmacy is often associated with complex drug interactions and additive drug toxicities. Furthermore, the incidence of adverse drug reactions (ADRs) is much higher in HIV/AIDS patients compared to non-HIV-infected patients. For instance, with sulfonamide agents, the recorded incidence of rash/fever/pruritus in HIV patients is between 50 and 80 percent, compared to approximately less than 5 percent in the general population. This incidence also exceeds that of non-HIV infected immunosuppressed patients. In HIV patients, the sulfa rash typically occurs at day 10 to 14, but may occur at any time (days to months).

PATHOGENESIS

Reasons for the increased incidence of drug reactions in HIV-infected patients have not been fully elucidated. It is speculated that as HIV disease progresses, the body's ability to detoxify drugs and their metabolites is decreased. For example, the acetylator status may change when a patient is acutely ill, resulting in increased formation of toxic metabolites. Furthermore, glutathione stores are depleted with disease progression, thus reducing the body's ability to scavenge and detoxify metabolites.

CLINICAL SIGNIFICANCE

Many individuals are on numerous medications to treat or prevent opportunistic infections in later stages of illness. (Refer to Appendix 1 for detailed information on specific drugs.) The occurrence of side effects can potentially complicate management because therapeutic options are often limited. Development of an ADR may require switching to another agent (which may be less efficacious or more toxic), or discontinuing therapy completely. Suboptimal management may be associated with increased morbidity or mortality.

For example, PCP is the most common opportunistic infection in AIDS patients, causing death in up to 25 percent of patients. After an initial episode, the spontaneous relapse rate with inadequate prophylaxis is approximately 35 percent at 6 months and 60 percent at 1 year; subsequent episodes are associated with higher mortality than the first pneumonia. Although TMP-SMX is considered to be the gold standard for both treatment and prevention of PCP, patients are often intolerant of this agent. Thus, second-line agents (which are less efficacious and potentially more toxic) need to be employed.

SYSTEMATIC APPROACH TO ASSESSING ADVERSE DRUG REACTIONS

When dealing with a suspected or potential adverse drug reaction, it is important to use a systemic approach in order to determine causality. It is necessary to identify the most likely causative agent, for two reasons: first, so that appropriate management measures may be undertaken, and second, so that other medications are not discontinued unnecessarily.

The following is a systematic approach to dealing with adverse drug reactions:

1. Diagnosis

   - Define the adverse event.
   - Differentiate between side effect and true allergy.

2. Chronology

   - Establish the time course of the ADR in relation to drug exposure.
   - Determine whether the ADR occurred before or after the drug was started.

3. *Differential diagnosis.* Consider alternative drug and nondrug causes for adverse event.

4. *Literature review.*

   - Are details consistent with prior reports of similar events associated with the drug in question?
   - How consistent are the clinical features of the case(s)?

5. *Therapeutic options.*

   - *Continue.*
     —What is the course of the ADR?
     —Is it transient, or will it worsen with continued exposure?
   - *Decrease dose.*
     —Is the ADR dose-related?
     —Will a lower dose still be effective therapeutically?
   - *Is desensitization possible?*
     —How severe was the reaction?
     —What is the mechanism?
     —Are there protocols available? (See Appendix 3.)
     —What is the urgency of the situation? Is there time to prepare and institute a desensitization regimen?
   - *Change drug.*
     —Are other equally efficacious therapeutic agents available?
     —What is the risk of cross-reactivity (e.g., 30 percent cross-reactivity between sulfonamides and dapsone)?
   - *Add a drug to treat the ADR.* Consider additional cost, inconvenience, and potential drug interactions, as well as side effects of added agent.

- *Discontinue drug.*
  —What is the drug being used for?
  —How necessary is it to continue treatment?

6. Confirmative testing. Is rechallenge feasible (e.g., for TMP-SMX, rechallenge is contraindicated with a past history of anaphylaxis or Stevens–Johnson syndrome)?

Suggested Readings

Bayard PJ, Berger TG, Jacobson MA. Drug hypersensitivity reactions and human immunodeficiency virus disease. J AIDS 1992;5:1237–57.

Carr A, Cooper DA, Penny R. Allergic manifestations of human immunodeficiency virus (HIV) infection. J Clin Immunol 1991; 11:55–64.

Harb GE, Jacobson MA. Human immunodeficiency virus infection: does it increase susceptibility to adverse drug reactions? Drug Safety 1993;9:1–8.

Koopmans PP, van der Ven A, Vree TB, van der Meer J. Pathogenesis of hypersensitivity reactions to drugs in patients with HIV infection: allergic or toxic? AIDS 1995;9: 217–22.

■ DRUG INTERACTIONS IN HIV PATIENTS

Michelle Foisy, Pharm.D.

Alice Tseng, Pharm.D.

HIV patients often need to take many medications on a regular basis, especially during the later stages of their illness. Prescribing drugs can often be difficult because of issues related to both the HIV disease itself, as well as the other agents a patient may already be taking. In other words, *drug–disease, drug–drug,* and *drug–food* interactions need to be considered when selecting a particular drug, dose, or route of administration. This is important because of the potential consequences of drug interactions (i.e., therapeutic efficacy or toxicity may be affected).

This part is divided into two sections. The first is a brief overview of the principles of drug interactions. The second part discusses the approach to management of potential drug interactions. A comprehensive list of drug–drug and drug–food interactions is provided in the accompanying tables.

PRINCIPLES OF DRUG INTERACTIONS

Drug interactions can be broken down into two basic categories, based on mechanism:

1. *Pharmacokinetic* interactions, which involve a change in the *amount* of drug in the body. The absorption, distribution, metabolism, or elimination of a drug may be affected.

2. *Pharmacodynamic* interactions, which involve a change in the *effect* of a drug on the body. These interactions may be additive, synergistic, or antagonistic, and are either desirable or undesirable, depending on whether the efficacy or toxicity profile is affected.

Both of these categories apply to drug interactions with a disease state, other drugs, or food.

Drug–Disease Considerations

HIV infection can result in physiologic changes, which in turn may affect drug dosing or response. For instance, patients may not be able to fully absorb oral medications because of changes in gastric pH, HIV enteropathy, or diarrhea due to concurrent opportunistic infections.

Because of their impaired immune system, HIV patients will often require chronic suppressive therapy after treatment of an acute illness. These patients may also respond differently to various medications; for example, there is a much higher incidence of allergic reactions to sulfonamides in HIV patients compared to noninfected patients (see "Adverse Drug Reactions in HIV Patients," earlier in this chapter, for further information). These factors are summarized in Table 8–15.

Drug–Drug Interactions

When certain combinations of drugs are given, they may affect each other kinetically or dynamically.

1. *Kinetic interactions.* When certain combinations of drugs are given together, the amount of one or both agents in the body may be altered. This is especially undesirable when an agent with a narrow therapeutic index is affected.

2. *Pharmacodynamic interactions.* Certain agents may have overlapping pharmacologic effects. This can be *desirable* if:

TABLE 8–15

Drug–Disease Considerations in HIV Patients

DRUG DOSING/ RESPONSE	HIV DISEASE CHANGES	EXAMPLES	CLINICAL SIGNIFICANCE/ IMPLICATIONS
Dosing Absorption	Achlorhydria	Drugs that require gastric pH for absorption (e.g., ketoconazole, itraconazole)	Possible ↓ efficacy; may need to ↑ doses or change to another agent
	Enteropathy, malabsorption	TB/MAC medications, potentially others	Consider measuring drug serum concentrations (if available) May need to change route of administration (e.g., PO to IV)
Distribution	↓ body weight (fat, muscle)	Agents with dose-related toxicities (e.g., TB, CMV medications) Erratic absorption with IM injection; may also be more painful to patient (↑ risk of needlestick injuries)	Adjust doses to actual patient body weight Consider route of administration
	↓ serum albumin	Phenytoin	Affects interpretation of serum levels

(Continued)

TABLE 8–15

Drug–Disease Considerations in HIV Patients (Continued)

DRUG DOSING/ RESPONSE	HIV DISEASE CHANGES	EXAMPLES	CLINICAL SIGNIFICANCE/ IMPLICATIONS
Metabolism, elimination	Hepatitis, biliary disease	Hepatotoxic agents	May need to change dose, interval, medication selection
	Nephropathy	Renally cleared drugs (e.g., aminoglycosides)	
Response Efficacy	↓ immune status	Treating TB	May take longer to achieve therapeutic effect
		Management of opportunistic infections	Often requires life-long therapy to treat or prevent disease
Toxicity	↑ incidence	Sulfonamides (see previous part on ADR)	May need to use alternative agent (perhaps less efficacious, more toxic)
	↑ sensitivity	Neuroleptics (see Chapter 10)	May need to use lower doses to avoid toxicity

- One is trying to *enhance clinical efficacy* by using agents with complementary mechanisms of action. For example, in vitro, the combination of zidovudine plus 3TC has a greater effect on suppressing HIV viral load than either agent alone.

- One is trying to *reduce patient toxicity.* For example, a documented side effect of isoniazid is peripheral neuropathy; the concurrent administration of pyridoxine has been shown to decrease the incidence of this side effect.

However, certain combinations of agents may be *undesirable* if:

- The *risk of therapeutic failure is increased* by using agents that antagonize each other's mechanism of action, for example, giving a bacteriocidal agent (e.g., amphotericin B) plus a bacteriostatic agent (e.g., fluconazole).

- The *risk of toxicity is increased* by using agents with overlapping side effect profiles. For example, the risk of hematotoxicity is increased when zidovudine is administered concurrently with ganciclovir.

These principles are summarized in Table 8–16. Information regarding specific drug–drug and drug–food combinations is given in Appendices 3 and 4.

APPROACH TO MANAGEMENT OF DRUG INTERACTIONS

1. *Verify the existence of an interaction.*

   - How was the interaction described? Was it in a retrospective observation, case report, or a controlled pharmacokinetic trial?
   - Can the data be applied to your patient population?
     —What patient population was the interaction observed in?
     —Are they representative of the type of patients you are dealing with (e.g., HIV versus non-HIV infected; asymptomatic HIV patient with CD4 >500 versus AIDS patient with CD4 <50)?
     —Were the drugs and dosages similar to those used in your daily practice?
   - Time frame (e.g., enzyme induction/inhibition): has the interaction already occurred?
     —Generally with enzyme inhibition, the interaction is seen within 1 to 2 days; likewise, when the offending

TABLE 8-16

Drug-Drug Interactions in HIV Patients

KINETIC/ DYNAMIC	DRUG-DRUG EFFECTS	EXAMPLES	CLINICAL SIGNIFICANCE/ IMPLICATIONS
Kinetic			
Absorption	Changes in pH	Didanosine/ketoconazole or itraconazole	$\downarrow$ absorption $\rightarrow$ $\downarrow$ efficacy
	Dissolution, chelation	Didanosine/ciprofloxacin or tetracycline	$\downarrow$ rifampin absorption ($\downarrow$ efficacy)
	Drug/food (see Appendix 4)	Ketoconazole/rifampin	$\uparrow$ absorption ($\uparrow$ efficacy/toxicity?)
		Atovaquone/fatty meal	
Distribution	Binding displacement	Phenytoin/TMP-SMX	$\uparrow$ phenytoin concentrations ($\uparrow$ risk toxicity)
Metabolism	Enzyme induction	Rifampin/ketoconazole	$\downarrow$ ketoconazole concentration ($\uparrow$ risk breakthrough fungal infection)
	Enzyme inhibition	Rifabutin/fluconazole or clarithromycin	$\uparrow$ rifabutin concentrations, $\uparrow$ risk uveitis
Elimination	Competition or inhibition	Amphotericin B/flucytosine	$\downarrow$ clearance of flucytosine $\rightarrow$ $\uparrow$ toxicity

Dynamic		
Efficacy	Synergism	Potential ↑ therapeutic effect
	Antagonism	Potential ↓ therapeutic effect
	Zidovudine/lamivudine	
	Amphotericin B/fluconazole	
Toxicity	Additive, synergistic effects	↑ risk of toxicity
	Drugs with overlapping toxicities, e.g., zidovudine/ganciclovir (↑ risk hematotoxicity)	May need to ↓ dose(s) or change drug(s)
	Didanosine/pentamidine (↑ risk pancreatitis)	

agent is removed, the effect should resolve within a similar time frame (e.g., fluconazole–phenytoin).

—Since most enzyme inducers reach steady state at 10 to 14 days, the full impact of the interaction may not be evident immediately; similarly, once the offending agent is removed, the effect will take a few weeks to resolve (e.g., rifampin–oral contraceptives).

2. *Clinical significance of the interaction.*

  ▪ Do the agents involved have a narrow therapeutic index (e.g., dose-related efficacy/toxicity of drug)?

  ▪ Is there risk of therapeutic failure or resistance developing?

    —What is the agent being used for (disease state being treated)?

    —What are the consequences of therapeutic failure or resistance (e.g., increased morbidity, mortality)?

  ▪ Is the patient at increased risk of experiencing side effects?

3. *Evaluate available therapeutic alternatives.* These will depend upon both the mechanism of the interaction and the clinical significance of the interaction.

  ▪ Space dosing times (e.g., ciprofloxacin and ddI).

  ▪ Alter dose (increase/decrease) (e.g., decrease or hold zidovudine while giving induction ganciclovir).

  ▪ Change agent (e.g., change ketoconazole to fluconazole when using rifampin).

  ▪ Add another agent to manage the effect of an interaction (e.g., administer G-CSF to counteract neutopenia induced by combined zidovudine and ganciclovir).

Suggested Readings

Burger DM, Meenhorst PL, Koks CHW, Beijen JH. Drug interactions with zidovudine. AIDS 1993;7:445–60.

Gillum JG, Israel DS, Polk RE. Pharmacokinetic drug interactions with antimicrobial agents. Clin Pharmacokinet 1993;25:450–82.

Lee BL, Safrin S. Interactions and toxicities of drugs used in patients with AIDS. Clin Infect Dis 1992;14:773–9.

Morris DJ. Adverse effects and drug interactions of clinical importance with antiretroviral drugs. Drug Safety 1994;10:281–91.

Psychiatric and Psychosocial Issues

PSYCHIATRIC DISORDERS IN HIV-INFECTED INDIVIDUALS

Mark H. Halman, M.D., F.R.C.P.C.

Management of psychiatric disorders in patients with HIV disease must include assessment of a wide range of predisposing, precipitating, and perpetuating factors, including premorbid primary psychiatric disorders, substance-related disorders, consequences of HIV central nervous system infection, organic sequelae of advanced HIV disease, and the medications used to treat HIV disease as well as the psychological impact of a life-threatening illness. As the contribution of organic factors to mental status changes will increase with the advancement of systemic illness, psychiatric evaluation must consider the clinical stage of the patient as well as laboratory markers of immune dysfunction and viral burden. The intersection of such a wide array of complex factors necessitates careful patient evaluation, consideration of multiple diagnoses, and interventions targeted to specific diagnostic criteria. This section will consider the most common psychiatric and neuropsychiatric disorders that complicate HIV disease and focus on the evaluation and psychopharmacologic management of these disorders. Subsequent chapters will deal with counseling and psychotherapeutic treatments.

HIV-1-ASSOCIATED COGNITIVE/MOTOR COMPLEX

The term *HIV-1-associated cognitive/motor complex* (HACM) was adopted by the American Academy of Neurology as a consensus nomenclature for the neurodegenerative disorder associated with HIV-1 infection. Other terms include *HIV-1 subacute encephalitis, HIV-1 encephalopathy, AIDS dementia complex,* and *dementia due to HIV disease.* HACM is the term used throughout this section and is the preferred clinical nomenclature.

HACM is characterized by cognitive, affective, behavioral, and motor dysfunction. Domains of cognitive deficits include fine motor speed and control, concentration and attention, executive function, and visuospatial performance. Patients describe poor attention, short-term memory loss, the need to write things down, a general slowing down of function, word-finding difficulties, and difficulty with sequential tasks, and describe that activities that were once automatic now require effortful concentration for successful completion, suggesting impairment of implicit memory. Impairments of higher cortical functions, such as aphasia and agnosia, are rare, except in end-stage disease. Behaviorally, patients commonly report apathy, loss of motivation, anergia, and fatigue, with social withdrawal commonly developing as a consequence. Although depressed mood may frequently coexist, the behavioral changes can also occur in the absence of the qualitative affective component of sadness. Mania and hypomania are less common but have been reported in association with advanced systemic HIV disease, as has new-onset psychosis. Motor changes include psychomotor slowing, clumsiness, unsteadiness of gait, and deterioration of handwriting. The criteria for diagnosis of HACM are outlined in Table 9–1.

The longitudinal course of progressive HACM is characterized by a slowing down process in the domains of cognition, affect, behavior, and motor functions, progressing slowly over time. Intercurrent infection or metabolic disturbances may transiently worsen the severity of cognitive dysfunction or increase the slope of the deterioration course. Departures from a typical longitudinal course, or presentation of unexpected symptoms, should prompt investigations for causes other than, or in addition to, HACM to account for the mental status changes. Examples of departures include very rapid deterioration in course, focal neurologic findings, seizures, psychosis, or mania. Over time the progression of deficits leads to greater impairment of overall function, with impact on work and activities of daily living. Patients with minimal cognitive dysfunction do not follow a progressive course of deterioration but rather exhibit a stable deficit over time with no deterioration or only mild transient worsening during periods of intercurrent insult. It remains unclear if

TABLE 9–1

American Academy of Neurology Criteria for HIV-1-Associated Cognitive/Motor Complex

1. Acquired abnormality in at least two of the following cognitive abilities (present for ≥1 month):

Attention/concentration	Speed of processing
Abstraction/reasoning	Visuospatial skills
Memory learning	Speech/language

   a) Decline verified by history and mental status examination. When possible, history should be obtained by an informant, and examination supplemented by neuropsychological testing.

   b) Cognitive dysfunction causing impairment of work or activities of daily living; impairment not attributable solely to severe systemic illness.

2. At least one of the following:

   a) Acquired abnormality in motor function or performance verified by physical examination, neuropsychological tests, or both.

   b) Decline in motivation or emotional control or change in social behavior, characterized by any of the following:

   > apathy, intertia, irritability, emotional lability, or new-onset impaired judgment, characterized by socially inappropriate behavior or disinhibition

3. Absence of clouding of consciousness during a period long enough to establish the presence of #1.

4. Evidence of another etiology, including active CNS opportunistic infections or malignancy, psychiatric disorders (e.g., depressive disorders), active substance abuse, or acute or chronic substance withdrawal, must be ruled out by history, physical and psychiatric examination, and appropriate laboratory and radiologic tests.

AAN Working Group: Nomenclature and research case definitions for neurologic manifestations of HIV-1 infection. Neurology 41: 778-85.

minimal neurocognitive disorder and progressive HACM are two distinct entities or a single continuous entity differentiated only by severity.

Severity of functional impact of HACM can be assessed using the Memorial Sloan-Kettering (MSK) clinical rating system, based on clinical history and neurologic examination, outlined in Table 9–2. Patients with minimal- or mild-severity ADC (MSK stages 0.5 or 1) experience cognitive deficits which do not adversely impact upon daily social and occupational functioning and hence do not meet impairment criteria for dementia, but are experiencing a neurologic complication of HIV infection that some inves-

TABLE 9-2

Memorial Sloan-Kettering Clinical Staging System for ADC

ADC STAGE		CHARACTERISTICS
Stage 0	(normal)	Normal mental and motor function.
Stage 0.5	(equivocal)	Either minimal or equivocal symptoms of cognitive or motor dysfunction characteristic of HIV-1-associated cognitive/motor complex, or mild signs (snout response, slowed extremity movements), but without impairment of work or capacity to perform activities of daily living (ADLs). Gait and strength
Stage 1	(mild)	Unequivocal evidence (symptoms, signs, neuropsychological test performance) of functional intellectual or motor impairment characteristic of HIV-1-associated cognitive/motor complex, but able to perform all but the more demanding aspects of work or ADLs. Can walk without assistance.
Stage 2	(moderate)	Cannot walk or maintain the more demanding ADLs, but able to perform basic ADLs of self care. Ambulatory, but may require a single prop.
Stage 3	(severe)	Major intellectual incapacity (cannot follow news or personal events, cannot sustain complex conversation, considerable slowing of all output) or motor disability (cannot walk unassisted, requiring walker or personal support, usually with slowing and clumsiness of arms as well).
Stage 4	(end stage)	Nearly vegetative. Intellectual and social comprehension and output are at a rudimentary level. Nearly or absolutely mute. Parapetic or paraplegic with double incontinence (urinary and bowel).

Price RW and Brew DJ. Memorial Sloan-Kettering clinical staging of AIDS dementia complex. J Infect Dis *1988;158:1079-83.*

tigators have termed *minimal neurocognitive disorder*. A diagnosis of dementia, which implies both global cognitive deficits and significant impact on function, is consistent with MSK stage ≥2.

Prevalence estimates for HACM MSK stage ≥2 among patients with HIV disease are 15 to 19 percent, with an annual incidence of 3 to 7 percent. Approximately 4 percent of HIV-infected patients present with HACM MSK stage ≥2 as their AIDS-defining diagnosis. Lifetime prevalence of minimal neurocognitive disorder has been reported to be as high as 40 to 60 percent of HIV-infected patients, indicating that not all patients with minimal neurocognitive disorder progress to a full dementia syndrome. The prevalence of cognitive dysfunction secondary to HIV infection parallels the progression of systemic HIV disease with deficits uncommon in asymptomatic HIV infection and more common in patients with an AIDS-defining condition. Similar patterns of cognitive deficit have been demonstrated across HIV infection acquisition risk factor group (i.e., similar patterns have been demonstrated among both homosexual/bisexual men and injection drug users).

Diagnosis of HACM is based upon a suggestive history and neurologic and psychiatric examinations. There is no single investigation, taken alone, upon which the diagnosis of HACM can be made. Neuropsychological testing, anatomic brain imaging, cerebrospinal fluid (CSF) examination, and blood work are used to support the findings of clinical examination and to exclude other causes of CNS dysfunction.

Routine investigational blood work includes hemoglobin, glucose, electrolytes, calcium, albumin, magnesium, vitamin B_{12}, thyroid stimulating hormone (TSH), and serologic testing for syphilis. Other blood work may be done if metabolic disturbance or endocrinopathies are suggested on clinical examination. If psychoactive substance-related disorders are suspected, a drug screen should be done. Levels of psychoactive drugs, including anticonvulsants, sedatives, narcotics, anticholinergics, antidepressants, and alcohol, should be measured if intoxication is suspected.

Anatomic brain imaging techniques are most useful in detecting other causes of CNS dysfunction, such as mass or vascular lesions due to *Toxoplasma* encephalitis, lymphoma, or stroke, which may complicate the course of HIV-1 disease. Radiologic correlation with clinical staging of HACM alone or with neuropsychological performance has been limited. Brain imaging techniques are neither reliably sensitive to detect early changes nor do they show a high degree of specificity in clinical staging. The most common finding on imaging is cerebral atrophy and ventricular enlargement on both computed tomography (CT) or magnetic resonance imaging (MRI). MRI may also detect patchy T_2-weighted white matter lesions and is more sensitive than CT in detecting regional atrophic changes, such as in the basal ganglia. A patient presenting with new-onset cognitive dysfunction should have a head CT to rule out detectable lesions and to establish a baseline image, but the limitations in specificity and predictive value of the findings must be acknowledged.

Single photon emission computed tomography (SPECT) remains a research tool at present, as findings appear to inconsistently correlate with measures of HACM severity. A pattern of multifocal perfusion defects with a frontal lobe predominance may be an indicator of HIV CNS infection, but its clinical usefulness is limited by its lack of specificity. An identical SPECT pattern is seen in non-HIV-infected patients with cocaine dependence and a similar pattern of perfusion defects is seen in HIV-infected patients without neurocognitive abnormalities. Initial studies with positron emission tomography (PET) have found a pattern of subcortical hypermetabolism and cortical hypometabolism in patients with early HACM, whereas those with advanced HACM showed subcortical hypometabolism. This also remains a research tool only.

Electroencephalography (EEG) may show mild nonspecific slowing, but contributes little to the diagnostic evaluation unless a seizure disorder is clinically suspected.

CSF examination may show pleocytosis, elevated IgG, oligoclonal bands, and increased protein, all of which are nonspecific and do not correlate well with clinical severity. The major use of the CSF examination is to exclude other causes of mental status changes, including opportunistic infections, tumors, and syphilis.

Neuropsychological testing is used to objectively document cognitive deficits and characterize cognitive function, interpreted within the clinical context. Tests of attention, memory, motor speed, and cognitive flexibility that incorporate time pressure and problem solving are sensitive to HIV-related cognitive deficits. Baseline testing with longitudinal follow-up provides a means to monitor for progression of cognitive dysfunction and gives a better measure of clinical progression than cross-sectional testing alone. Longitudinal testing is also helpful in evaluating response to treatment interventions. Testing can also assist in planning cognitive rehabilitation or behavioral interventions used in treatment.

Screening tests, in conjunction with clinical interview, may be useful to indicate which patients need a more extensive neuropsychological evaluation. The AIDS clinical trials group (ACTG) uses a battery incorporating the Timed Gait, Grooved Pegboard, Finger Tapping, and Digit Symbol tests. The Multicenter AIDS Cohort Study (MACS) has used computer-based reaction time screening measures. The Folstein mini-mental state examination (MMSE), relying on tests that measure functions rarely impaired until advanced stages of HACM, is not sensitive to mild dysfunction and hence is not useful as a screening tool in this disorder. A screening examination should incorporate tests of attention, short-term memory, frontal executive function, and motor speed.

HACM must be differentiated from, or may coexist with, other causes of cognitive dysfunction in HIV-infected patients, which can be broadly categorized as follows:

- Infectious disorders: both intracranial and systemic, including opportunistic infections as immune dysfunction progresses.

- Metabolic disorders: endocrinopathies and vitamin deficiencies.

- Vascular disorders: including anemia, hypotension, and vasculitidies.

- Seizure disorders.

- Intracranial mass occupying lesions including neoplasms.

- Drug intoxications and substance-related disorders, including withdrawal states and medication side effects.

- Head trauma.

- Primary psychiatric disorders.

Differentiating HACM from a major depressive disorder is a common clinical difficulty. The criteria for major depressive disorder are outlined in the discussion of depressive disorders, and the overlap of symptoms is high. Frequently the two disorders coexist and both need to be appropriately treated. The presence of apathy, amotivation, and anergia along with cognitive deficits consistent with those outlined in the criteria for HACM, in the absence of a qualitative subjective sense of sadness, is more suggestive of HACM or consequences of advanced systemic HIV disease than a major depressive episode and should lead the investigations in the direction of an organic etiology. Sometimes a therapeutic trial of antidepressants is necessary to distinguish the two disorders.

Antiretroviral agents are considered first line therapy in treating HACM. Zidovudine (AZT) has been shown to improve neuropsychological performance over the short-term, and may have a protective effect in delaying the progression of cognitive deficits. The long-term impact of antiretrovirals on the course of HACM remains largely unknown, as does the timing of treatment initiation and optimum dosage. All antiretrovirals may be effective in treating HACM but zidovudine may be most effective, as it has the greatest penetration of the blood–brain barrier. Studies demonstrating efficacy of zidovudine on neuropsychological outcomes found very high doses (2000 mg) to be most effective, but such doses are not clinically manageable for most patients and optimal dosing needs to balance the demonstrated benefit of higher doses against the negative impact on quality of life.

Neuroprotective agents, designed to stop the progression of neuronal dysfunction, may be effective for HACM. The calcium channel antagonist nimodipine and the NMDA-glutamate antagonist memantine are currently under investigation but do not yet have a role in clinical treatment.

Symptomatic treatment of specific syndromes, including delirium, psychosis, depression, and manic disorders, warrant specific evaluation and management and are discussed in subsequent sections. Fatigue, apathy, anergia, amotivation, and dysphoria, as well as cognitive symptoms, including poor concentration, may respond to a trial of psychostimulants. Psychosocial support and cognitive retraining to minimize the functional impact of neuropsychological deficits need to be part of the treatment strategy. Ultimately, transfer to supervised housing may need to be considered.

Summary of Management of HACM

1. ***Establishment of the diagnosis.*** Is the course typical? Are the symptoms consistent with criteria? If not, investigate other causes of mental status changes as directed by clinical examination.

2. ***Establishment of the baseline of cognitive function.*** (At the Wellesley Hospital, comprehensive neuropsychological evaluation, including psychiatric assessment and

neuropsychological testing, is done through referral to the HIV psychiatry service.)

3. ***Treatment of brain HIV infection, the presumptive underlying condition.*** Is the patient on antiretroviral medication? Is the dosing maximized? If the patient is not on antiretrovirals, recommend initiation of zidovudine at standard dose of 600 mg/day. If the patient is on zidovudine, but has progressive cognitive deterioration, consider higher doses (800 to 1500 mg/day) titrated against side effects and negative impact on quality of life of higher doses of antiretrovirals. If higher doses of zidovudine cannot be tolerated, consider switching to other antiretroviral or combination therapy. Neuropsychological follow-up assessments can guide effectiveness of treatment interventions.

4. ***Treatment of neuronal deterioration.*** The use of neuroprotective agents are currently under research investigation and may represent a future clinical treatment option.

5. ***Symptomatic treatment of specific psychiatric conditions*** that may accompany advanced HACM, including delirium, major depression, mania, sleep disorder, and psychosis.

6. ***Symptomatic treatment of anergia, fatigue, amotivation, and inattention.*** Low-dose psychostimulants may specifically target these symptoms with an onset of action within the first 48 hours. Start with methylphenidate 5 mg at 08:00 on day 1. If there is no effect on target symptoms increase to 10 mg at 08:00 by day 3. If no effect is experienced by increasing to 20 mg by day 6 then discontinue treatment and switch to a similarly increasing trial of dextroamphetamine. If effect on target symptoms is noted, maintain at the dose that produced symptom relief. If patient notes that symptoms improve after 08:00 dose but reemerge later in the day, a second dose, usually half the 08:00 dose, can be added at 11:00. Dosing after 12:00 noon will usually interfere with nighttime sleep. Daily doses above 40 mg should not be used. Patients need to be informed of the addictive potential of stimulants and physicians should maintain judicious prescribing habits to mitigate against nonjudicious dose escalation. Physicians should also be aware that although stimulants have been demonstrated to be effective in open-label trials and are clinically considered effective they have not been evaluated in randomized double-blind

placebo-controlled studies and HACM is not an approved indication for their use.

DELIRIUM

Patients with advanced systemic disease and HACM are at high risk for delirium, which is the most frequent neuropsychiatric complication in hospitalized patients with AIDS. The cause of delirium is usually multifactorial, commonly reflecting an organic cause superimposed upon a brain left vulnerable to insult by predisposing brain HIV infection. The primary goal in management of delirium is the identification and treatment of the underlying factors contributing to mental status changes, outlined above. Delirium is characterized by a disturbance in consciousness with reduced ability to focus, sustain or shift attention, with accompanying disturbance of cognition and/or perception. It generally develops rapidly over a short period of time and follows a fluctuating course over the day. Investigations, including EEG, anatomic brain imaging, CSF examination, and blood work must be guided by clinical examination.

Antipsychotic medication is used for symptomatic relief and may be necessary to control agitation and assist in resolving confusion. Patients with HIV-1 disease are at increased risk for extrapyramidal side effects secondary to the use of high-potency antipsychotics such as haloperidol, so the minimum antipsychotic dose necessary to control target symptoms should be used. Target symptoms, including agitation, sleep disturbance, confusion, and dangerous behavior, should be identified and the effect of the antipsychotic on those symptoms noted. Treatment should begin with haloperidol 0.5 mg and target symptoms reassessed in 30 minutes. If symptoms are not improved a dose of 1.0 mg should be given. Frequent reassessment and careful titration will allow symptom control with minimum necessary dosage. Most patients will respond to a daily dose equivalent of 0.5 to 5.0 mg but higher doses may be necessary and must be used as dictated by the clinical situation, recognizing that untreated delirium has considerable associated morbidity and mortality. Haloperidol dosing is equivalent for all routes of administration (IV, IM, PO) but is most rapid in onset when given by IV dosing if allowed by clinical situation and institutional policy. Anticholinergic medications used to protect against the development of extrapyramidal side effects from antipsychotics may worsen a delirium and routine use should be avoided, though they can be used if a dystonic reaction occurs. Benzodiazepenes should not be used as a single agent in the treatment of delirium, but lorazepam may be a useful adjunct to antipsychotics, particularly with very agitated patients in whom achieving sedation is an important target symptom. In emergency situations where untreated delirium may pose a threat to the safety of the patient or the treatment team, mechanical restraint may be used with clear targeted behavioral objectives to bring the situation under safe medical control and to allow necessary medical stabilization.

MAJOR DEPRESSIVE DISORDERS

Depressed mood occurs in almost all patients at some point in the course of HIV disease but should be distinguished from major depression, a clinical syndrome made up of a constellation of symptoms, meeting specific diagnostic criteria and requiring specific treatment interventions, which although common, is not a naturally expected consequence of HIV disease. Major depressive disorders are commonly underdiagnosed, and frequently rationalized as a reasonable response to developing a fatal illness. Failure to diagnose and treat a major depressive disorder may significantly add to the morbidity experienced by the patient over the course of illness.

Community-based cohort studies report current rates of major depression at 4 to 18 percent in gay/bisexual men at early stages of HIV disease and 35 percent in infected injection drug users. Longitudinal follow-up studies indicate that the prevalence of major depression increases with the progression of systemic HIV disease and immunologic dysfunction. This may be accounted for by both increased psychological reactions to advancing illness as well as CNS effects of systemic HIV disease, and sequelae of HACM. These high rates of major depression in advanced HIV disease/AIDS are similar to those seen in other neurologic disorders that affect the subcortical structures, such as Parkinson's and Huntington's disease. Endocrinologic and metabolic disturbances, including adrenocortical insufficiency, hypothyroidism, euthyroid-sick syndrome, vitamin B_{12} deficiency, protein and calorie malnutrition, and decreased free testosterone levels, which may all complicate advanced stages of HIV-1 disease, may also contribute to depressive symptomatology. Psychosocial stressors associated with major depression in HIV-infected patients include unemployment, lower education, unresolved grief, and past history of mood disorders and substance-related disorders.

The diagnosis of a major depression episode is made using the criteria set forth in the DSM-IV. These include the presence of five of nine criteria, persisting for at least 2 weeks, with at least one of the criteria being either persistently depressed mood or loss of interest or pleasure in all, or almost all, activities. The other symptoms include disorder of sleep, appetite, psychomotor retardation or agitation, fatigue or loss of energy, feelings of worthlessness or excessive guilt, diminished capacity to concentrate, and recurrent thoughts of suicide or a persistent desire to be dead. Clearly, many of the neurovegatative somatic symptoms of major depression (decreased sleep, appetite, energy, concentration, and psychomotor retardation) overlap with symptoms of progressive HIV disease, thus complicating the diagnosis. The presence of somatic symptoms without the subjective affective experiences (depressed mood, loss of pleasure and interest, thoughts of guilt and worthlessness, desire to be dead) argues against the diagnosis of major depression and should prompt investigations for other causes, including endocrinopathies, HACM, and other conditions associated with advanced systemic illness. When the subjective affective symptoms are present, along with the somatic symptoms, it is usually futile to attempt to attribute the cause of the somatic symptoms to either major depression or systemic illness and management should be directed toward both treating the presumptive major depressive episode and ruling out other contributing factors of advanced systemic disease. A careful history of temporal relationships between the onset of depressed mood, specific neurovegatative somatic symptoms, and changes in systemic disease and medications as well as the patient's personal and familial premorbid history of major depression may help to clarify the diagnosis. Finally, the subjective mood quality may be a useful guide, with patients having major depression more commonly experiencing a sense of sadness and those with advanced systemic illness and/or HACM experiencing a mood quality characterized by boredom and apathy.

Antidepressant medications are effective in the treatment of a major depressive disorder. In general, mood disorders complicated by coexistent HACM, substance-related disorders, personality disorders, and/or advanced systemic illness are less responsive than primary uncomplicated mood disorders but still show significant degrees of treatment response, particularly when coexistent factors are also managed. Baseline laboratory tests should include complete blood cell count (CBC), electrolytes, glucose, liver function tests, TSH, vitamin B_{12}, serologic testing for syphilis, and electrocardiogram in patients over 40, or with evidence of HIV-related cardiomyopathy, when heterocyclic antidepressants are being considered. In men with advanced HIV disease, free testosterone levels should be measured if a hypogonadal state is clinically suspected, as this can be readily corrected with intramuscular anabolic steroids, which may significantly improve mood and energy states.

Antidepressants are generally well tolerated and efficacious in depressed HIV-infected patients and used safely even in severely ill patients. In general, with progression of symptomatic disease, patients experience more side effects and are less able to tolerate higher doses of antidepressants and as such may be less treatment responsive. As a general rule, antidepressants should be initiated at low doses and the dosage increased slowly, titrated against side effects. Antidepressants are chosen based on past treatment response and side effect profile.

Selective serotonin reuptake inhibitors (SSRIs), including fluoxetine, paroxetine, fluvoxamine, and sertraline, are all generally effective for HIV-related major depression and are well tolerated even in patients with advanced HIV disease, with rates of treatment response reported between 57 and 83 percent. Cited limitations to full response have been advanced systemic disease, lower CD4 lymphocyte count, and increased number of medications presumably due to drug interactions that increase the intolerability of superimposed side effects. In general, SSRIs are most effective in treatment of moderate severity outpatient depressions and can bring significant relief and improvement of quality of life.

Recommended treatment dose of fluoxetine and paroxetine is 20 mg daily, usually as a single AM dosing. Patients should start at half dose (i.e., 10 mg daily) for 1 week to diminish the side effects associated with treatment initiation and then increase to 20 mg if tolerated. Treatment response is usually seen in the first 4 to 6 weeks and treatment nonresponse should not be diagnosed until week 8. If there is no response, or only limited response by week 6 to 8, and the patient can tolerate higher doses, the dose should be increased by increments of 10 mg/day every 2 to 3 weeks to a maximum of 40 mg of paroxetine and 60 mg of fluoxetine. The majority of patients will respond to 20 to 40 mg and if no response is seen at that time psychiatric consultation should be sought. Treatment response is characterized by decreased agitation, increased sense of calm, improvement of somatic symptoms, resolution of sleep disturbance, and improving mood quality over a course of 3 to 6 weeks. Fluvoxamine is initiated at 50 mg qhs, and increased over a few days to an average effective dose of 100 mg BID, with maximal dosing being 150 mg BID. Sertraline is started at 50 mg qhs and although there is no established dose response curve, underdosing with sertraline can be a reason for nonresponse and the dose should be increased more rapidly than with paroxetine or fluoxetine, up to a maximal daily dose of 200 mg. All the SSRIs share similar side effect profiles, with gastrointestinal effects, nausea, headache, agitation, and anxiety being common in the first week to 10 days of treatment, after which the symptoms tend to subside without the need for dose reduction. These side effects tend to recur for a period of 7 to 10 days also following dose increase and then subside again with time. Decreased libido, erectile dysfunction, ejaculatory delay and anorgasmia are dose-dependent side effects of all SSRIs, and may be dose-limiting for many. Both fluoxetine and paroxetine are stimulating and should not be taken at bedtime as they may interfere with sleep. Even taken in the morning, sleep may remain disturbed and other strategies to assist with sleep disturbance should be implemented (see the discussion of sleep disorders). Both fluoxetine and paroxetine are highly protein bound and may raise the free level of other medications (e.g. warfarin) by displacement, necessitating dosage alteration. Finally, all SSRIs may contribute to weight loss, which can be problematic in this patient population and may necessitate drug discontinuation.

Heterocyclic antidepressants (HCAs) have also been found to be effective in HIV-infected patients, with response rates of 70 to 75 percent and with no adverse effects on markers of immune function. In general, HCAs are equally effective as SSRIs in the treatment of moderate outpatient depressions but carry more side effects, which may limit compliance or attainment of maximal therapeutic dosage. HCAs may be more effective in severe depressions, particularly those requiring inpatient admission. Nortriptyline and desipramine are two prototype HCAs that are generally well tolerated and effective. Nortriptyline is sedating and thus very useful when sleep disturbance or agitation is prominent. Desipramine is less sedating and in some patients may have a stimulating effect. Dosing regimens in patients with advanced systemic HIV disease will need to follow the start low, increase slowly model, whereas patients without systemic or CNS complications of HIV disease can be increased more quickly. In patients with more advanced disease, nortriptyline can be initiated at 10 mg daily at bedtime and increased by 10 mg every 2 to 3 days to an average therapeutic dose of 50 to 100 mg, titrated against side effects. In healthier patients dosing can begin at 25 mg and be increased by increments of 25 mg daily every 2 to 3 days to a maximum dosage of 150 mg. Serum nortriptyline levels in HIV-infected patients can be measured and are similar to standard therapeutic levels used in noninfected patients. Orthostatic hypotension is a troublesome side effect associated with HCAs and occurs frequently in patients with advanced HIV disease. It is mediated by the alpha-adrenergic antagonism associated with HCAs and is worsened in patients with autonomic neuropathy, dehydration, and muscle wastage. Patients need to be cautioned to change from lying to standing slowly to minimize the consequences of this side effect and to maintain their hydration status. Other side effects include dry mouth, blurred vision, constipation, urinary retention, and sexual dysfunction. Serum nortriptyline levels are not necessary for routine use, but should be used in patients who do not respond at average therapeutic doses, or in patients who develop dose limiting side effects at low doses.

In general, 60 to 75 percent of patients should have a treatment response to standard antidepressant therapy. Common reasons for nonresponse include underdosing, limitation of dose secondary to side effects, and noncompliance. Treatment regimens should be kept uncomplicated to maximize compliance and decrease potential for drug interactions. However, particularly in patients with advanced illness, in whom many targeted symptoms and conditions coexist and in whom maximal drug dosages may not be possible because of dose-limiting side effects, combination strategies may be utilized. These may include standard augmentation strategies in treatment refractory depression (SSRI/HCA + lithium carbonate or triiodothyronine; SSRI + low dose HCA [e.g., desipramine]), the addition of low-dose trazodone to an SSRI to specifically target sleep disturbance, or the addition of a low-dose stimulant, as outlined in the earlier discussion of HACM, in patients in whom an antidepressant (SSRI/HCA) may target the symptoms of depression but not the anergia, fatigue, and concentration difficulties associated with coexistent HACM.

All classes of antidepressants have the potential to induce a manic or hypomanic episode (see discussion of manic disorders for description). Patients at greatest risk of this side effect are those who have had a past history of mania or a past history of antidepressant-induced mania, and those with a strong family history of bipolar mood disorder (manic depressive disorder). In the absence of such a history, the chances of antidepressant-induced mania is low but still exists. Prior to starting antidepressant therapy all patients should be screened for a past history of mania and advised that antidepressant-induced mania is a potential side effect. If it is suspected that the patient has a predisposition to developing a manic episode, antidepressant therapy should not be commenced without a formal psychiatric evaluation. Other reasons to refer a patient with depression for psychiatric assessment includes differentiating depression with psychotic features, depression refractory to standard antidepressant treatment, depression complicated by prominent suicidal ideation and intent, and depression with coexistent HACM.

SUICIDE

Elevated suicide rates among persons with AIDS have been reported since the beginning of the epidemic, with the most common methods being drug overdose, firearms, and suffocation. The increased risk for suicide may be due to multiple factors, including premorbid psychopathology as well as the psychosocial morbidity associated with HIV disease. Homosexual youths and persons with substance-related disorders are at increased risk of suicide regardless of HIV serologic status. Factors associated with suicide in HIV-infected patients include the presence of a major depressive episode, substance-related disorders, alcohol intoxication, personality disorders, social isolation and the perception of poor social support, unemployment, HIV-related occupational problems, and poverty associated with illness, as well as a past history of suicide attempt. The period of the first 6 months following notification of HIV seropositivity and periods of progression of clinical disease and advancing immune dysfunction are associated with increased risk of suicide attempts.

Management includes the identification of patients at risk and treating underlying psychiatric disorders, particularly major depressive disorders, and substance-related disorders. A determination of the acuity of intervention must be made, based on the lethality potential of an active plan or intent, versus ideation or passive desire to be dead. New-onset suicidal ideation, representing a departure in previous coping style of the patient, should merit urgent consultation or action. Intervention, including psychiatric hospitalization, should be used to guarantee the patient's safety in order to treat any comorbid psychiatric disorders that may underlie the suicidality. In addition to pharmacologic management, the experience of talking about anticipated fears of future pain, emotional suffering, loss of autonomy, and loneliness can help the patient feel less isolated with his or her feelings and more able to maintain a connection with the human world.

MANIC DISORDERS

An acute manic episode is characterized by a period of abnormally elevated or irritable mood lasting at least 1 week and accompanied by at least three of the following: grandiosity and inflated self esteem, decreased need for sleep, increased talkativeness with pressured speech, racing thoughts, distractibility, increased goal-directed behavior or psychomotor agitation, and excessive involvement in pleasure-seeking activities that involve high potential for negative consequences (e.g., shopping sprees, sexual indiscretions). This episode leads to disturbance in function and often necessitates hospitalization to prevent a destructive outcome. A manic episode in an HIV-infected patient may be due to a primary bipolar mood disorder, secondary to a substance-related disorder, or secondary to an organic insult associated with HIV disease, including HACM, CNS opportunistic infections and tumors, and medication side effects. Although uncommon, cases of mania have been reported secondary to the use of zidovudine, corticosteroids, ganciclovir, ddI, and anabolic steroids. Cocaine and/or amphetamine-related disorders may also present as an acute manic episode. It is hypothesized that the etiology of this syndrome in HIV-infected patients reflects biological predisposition to bipolar disorders in association with the degree of brain insult secondary to HIV and other injurious causes. Patients who present early in the course of disease with little or no evidence of HACM likely have a stronger predisposition to manic disorders based on personal or family history. Manic patients with no past personal or family history of a mood disorder tend to present at more advanced stages of systemic disease and display more evidence of cognitive impairment associated with HACM.

Management of these patients can be quite complex, particularly in patients with evidence of coexistent HACM. It is important to remember that these patients can escalate rapidly and management must aim to ensure the safety of both the patient and those working with the patient. Patients with manic disorders tend to be highly distractible and often worsen with excessive stimulation. As such, patient contact should be clear and brief in a calm and secure environment devoid of distractions. Control of an escalating patient should be done in a manner to demonstrate that you can help the patient contain the dangerous behavior in a therapeutic and nonpunitive manner.

Standard pharmacotherapy for an acute manic episode includes the use of antipsychotics, benzodiazepenes, and lithium. Antipsychotics are the treatment of choice to rapidly contain an escalating patient, but in patients with advanced systemic disease and coexistent HACM, may be limited by the development of dose-limiting adverse side effects. Patients presenting earlier in the course of HIV disease without evidence of HACM tolerate antipsychotics similar to the general population. Antipsychotics should be initiated at low dose, titrating upward to gain control of target symptoms. Low-dose benzodiazepenes are effective adjunctive medication to help achieve a state of patient sedation. Typical initial dosing strategies in the emergency management of a patient without evidence of HACM would be haloperidol 5 mg and lorazepam 2 mg PO or IM and haloperidol 0.5 to 1 mg and lorazepam 1 mg in patients with evidence of HACM. Frequent reassessment of target symptoms is required until control of the situation is attained.

Once the emergency situation has been stabilized, evaluation for an underlying cause of the mental status change is necessary. The potential for organic contributors increases in patients with advanced systemic disease and HACM. Patients should undergo CBC, electrolytes, BUN, serum creatinine, creatinine clearance, TSH, electrocardiogram, and blood and urine drug screen. EEGs are frequently noncontributory but should be done if the episode is suggestive of a seizure disorder. A lumbar puncture is done if indicated by the clinical picture. Lithium is not used in the initial emergency management but is useful in the management of the acute episode as well as the prevention of future episodes in patients with a bipolar mood disorder. Lithium may be initiated at low doses (300 to 900 mg/day) and titrated upward to achieve clinical stabilization in the first week to 10 days, aiming for standard therapeutic levels of 0.6 to 1.2. In patients with advanced systemic HIV disease, dehydration, diarrhea, and poor oral intake necessitate careful monitoring of lithium levels. Lithium toxicity, including encephalopathy, may still develop despite normal therapeutic blood levels, presumably due to compromise of blood–brain barrier integrity.

In general, patients without HACM or advanced systemic HIV disease respond to lithium similar to the general population, but patients with HACM/advanced systemic disease frequently tolerate lithium quite poorly. Anticonvulsants, particularly valproic acid, may be an effective and well-tolerated alternative. A starting dose of 250 mg PO qhs is used and increased every 4 to 7 days by 250 mg daily, until symptomatic control is achieved. Liver function tests, hematologic parameters, particularly platelet count, and valproic acid levels need to be monitored. Valproic acid has been used safely with antiretrovirals and is known to raise zidovudine levels when the two drugs are coadministered (inhibition of cytochrome P450 system). Carbamazepine is also effective for mania, but may be problematic in patients with HIV disease because of increased risk for hematologic and dermatologic complications and may decrease zidovudine levels through induction of hepatic enzyme systems. As the mood-stabilizing agent (lithium, valproic acid, carbamazepine) begins to control the manic episode it is important to slowly decrease the antipsychotic medication to prevent the development of side effects associated with antipsychotic use, including dystonic reactions, parkinsonism, and akithisia. In all patients with advanced systemic HIV disease and presumptive coexistent HACM, investigations and management considerations described in the discussion of HACM should be initiated, including initiation of zidovudine. Psychostimulants should be discontinued during a manic episode, and if considered for use after the resolution of the manic episode for HACM-related symptoms, should be done under carefully monitored situations as the potential for inducing a future manic episode is high.

PSYCHOTIC DISORDERS

Psychosis is characterized by impairment of reality testing and is clinically manifested by delusions, persecutory ideation, thought disorder, and perceptual distortions, including hallucinations and illusions. New-onset psychosis in patients with HIV disease can be due to delirium, advanced HACM, complex partial seizures, and substance-related disorders. Psychosis may also be due to premorbid psychotic disorders, including schizophrenia and severe bipolar mood disorder.

Management includes those investigations outlined above for assessment of HACM. Emergency management and stabilization strategies involve similar principles to those outlined in the discussion of manic disorders. Antipsychotics (e.g., haloperidol, perphenazine, or loxapine) may all be effective in the management of psychosis. Patients with HACM, with no history of chronic mental illness, have been shown to have a higher than expected rate of extrapyramidal side effects with antipsychotic medications and may also be at increased risk for malignant neuroleptic syndrome. Thus antipsychotics must be initiated at lower doses with careful upward dose titration while monitoring for extrapyramidal side effects. An anticonvulsant (e.g., valproic acid) may be an important addition if hallucinations and delusions are accompanied by significant mood symptoms or if there is evidence that the psychosis is due to a seizure disorder. If psychosis is due to a primary psychotic disorder such as schizophrenia, maintenance antipsychotics will be the drugs of choice. With the progression of systemic HIV disease, the theoretical interaction among HIV brain effects, schizophrenia, and antipsychotic drug mechanisms suggests that patients may require smaller doses of antipsychotics to manage their psychotic symptoms and may be at higher risk of developing extrapyramidal side effects associated with antipsychotic use. Clozapine, which is increasingly being used for patients with schizophrenia, has not been studied in patients with HIV disease, but the potential for agranulocytosis, particularly in patients on medications with haematopoietic side effects such as zidovudine, as well as its capacity to lower the seizure threshold, precludes its use in this population. Psychostimulants should not be used in patients with psychotic disorders.

ANXIETY DISORDERS

Anxiety, similar to depression, is a frequently experienced emotion through the course of HIV disease and can present as a symptom of an adjustment disorder, may complicate a substance-related disorder, may coexist with a major depressive disorder, or may be a component of an anxiety disorder such as panic disorder or generalized anxiety disorder. The prevalence of anxiety disorders in HIV-infected individuals in community studies ranges from 2 to 18 percent in asymptomatic patients, 38 percent in patients with symptomatic but non-AIDS-defining condition, and 27 percent in patients with AIDS.

High levels of anxiety may occur in association with certain events in the course of HIV disease, including HIV serologic testing, onset of constitutional symptoms, initiation of antiretroviral treatment, first AIDS-defining condition, and hospitalization. The unpredictability associated with the progression of HIV disease, as well as the limited efficacy of treatment options, can all add to patients' anxiety. Panic attacks are discrete periods of intense fear, which begin abruptly, often without precipitant, and build over a 10-minute period, accompanied by at least four of the following symptoms: palpitations or increased heart rate, sweating, trembling, shortness of breath, choking, chest pain, nausea, dizziness, paresthesias, hot flashes, derealization, fear of going crazy or losing control, and fear of dying. Panic disorder is a condition in which panic attacks occur frequently and lead to a pattern of anticipatory anxiety over future attacks or avoidant behavior to escape having future attacks. Generalized anxiety disorder is the presence of anxiety on most days over at least a 6-month period accompanied by at least three of the following somatic symptoms: restlessness, fatiguability, difficulty concentrating, irritability, muscle tension, and sleep disturbance.

Cognitive behavioral therapy, dynamic psychotherapy both brief and longer term, and relaxation therapy may all be beneficial in the management of anxiety and represent the mainstay of treatment in helping the patient manage over the course of illness. Reduction of caffeine intake and provision of information and support are also important in the overall management. Pharmacotherapy is often necessary for discrete anxiety disorders. Antidepressants are first-line treatment option for the management of panic disorder and for anxiety associated with a major depressive episode, and should be used as outlined in the discussion of depression. Benzodiazepenes are extremely helpful when used acutely to enable the patient to regain psychological equilibrium. Benzodiazepenes cause physiological neuroadaptation in all patients and can lead to tolerance when used on a chronic basis. If tolerance leads to dose escalation, patients, particularly if they have coexistent HACM, become at increased risk for cognitive and motor side effects of benzodiazepenes. By contrast, psychological dependence and addiction are characterized by a drive state in which behavior is directed toward acquiring drug in a noncontrolled manner, often with serious negative consequences, and is found in only a minority of patients who frequently have comorbid substance-related or personality disorders. The potential for psychological dependence should not preclude the use of benzodiazepenes, as they represent an important intervention to reduce psychological distress for many patients. They do, however, need to be used in a judicious manner, with clear monitoring of target symptoms and an aim to use low doses for as short a period as possible. The different benzodiazepenes differ essentially in their pharmacokinetics, with short- to intermediate-half-life agents (lorazepam, oxazepam, clonazepam) being preferred over either long (diazepam, flurazepam) or ultra-short-half-life (triazolam) drugs. Coadministration of benzodiazepenes with zidovudine is safe and does not appear to affect the serum levels of either agent. Many patients find that they can manage their panic symptoms, generalized anxiety, or sleep disturbance with chronic low-dose benzodiazepenes without the need for dose escalation or the development of addictive behaviors and yet suffer significant relapse of anxiety symptoms when efforts are made to discontinue the benzodiazepenes. In such patients, chronic administration with clear monitoring of usage pattern may be the only option. In some patients with generalized anxiety disorder, buspirone 5 to 10 mg TID may be a helpful alternative to chronic benzodiazepeene, as it has little propensity for psychological dependence.

ADJUSTMENT DISORDERS

Adjustment disorders are common in the course of HIV disease. DSM-IV defines *adjustment disorders* as the development of emotional or behavioral symptoms in response to an identifiable stressor that causes marked distress in excess of what is expected from the stressor and leads to significant levels of impairment of social or occupational functioning. The stressor must have occurred within 3 months of the reaction and the symptoms not persist longer than 6 months. Common precipitants include HIV testing; disclosure of serologic status; progression of illness; illness of a partner, friend, or relative; decisions regarding treatment options; and couple-, family-, and child-related problems. Frequently multiple stressors exist and the disturbance becomes chronic as the patient adjusts and responds to overlapping and at times endless stressors. Patients can manifest different responses to stressors, including effects of depression, anxiety, and anger, as well as disturbances of behavior such as withdrawal or violating conduct.

The hallmark of treatment for adjustment disorders is counseling and psychotherapy. The treatment focus should be time limited, as the expectation is a resolution of the acute disturbance as the stressor resolves and the patient's equilibrium is regained. In HIV disease, in which many patients are contending with their own illness as well as living in a community dealing with multiple bereavements and loss, the temptation exists to understand all psychiatric disturbance as an adjustment disorder in response to chronic exposure to stressors. Frequently adjustment disorder is overdiagnosed to the exclusion of identifying a major psychiatric syndrome as symptoms are rationalized on the basis of the stressors that exist. This approach erroneously presumes that all people respond similarly to stressors and fails to appreciate the differences in situational factors, individual coping styles, and premorbid factors that shape people and predispose them to developing psychiatric morbidity. If a patient's symptoms persist or they develop a symptom complex consistent with another major psychiatric disorder, such as major depressive disorder, panic disorder, or generalized anxiety disorder, those diagnoses should be made and appropriate treatment interventions initiated.

Psychotherapy is frequently combined with pharmacotherapy in the acute situation. Psychotherapy needs to involve a flexible approach, incorporating psychoeducation and education about illness and treatment choices, and aiming to help the patient to restore function and emotional stability. It also involves allowing the ventilation of emotions, provision of support and information assisting in clarifying thoughts and arguments involved in decision making, and helping patients to access resources. Anxiety, agitation, and sleep disturbance are acute symptoms commonly experienced by many patients. A short course, 2 to 4 weeks of low doses of benzodiazepenes, can be very helpful while the patient stabilizes and begins to access support services.

SLEEP DISORDERS

Sleep complaints occur in the majority of patients with HIV disease at some point over the course of illness.

Examination should aim to identify and treat any coexistent psychiatric disorders and contributing organic factors. Primary sleep disorders have been reported in asymptomatic HIV-seropositive patients as well as patients with advanced systemic disease, with alteration in sleep architecture presumably resulting from either HIV CNS infection, secondary to host immune response to HIV infection or secondary to medications associated with the treatment of HIV disease including ddI, zidovudine, and acyclovir. Sleep complaints are often a symptom of associated psychiatric disorders such as major depressive episode, delirium, psychosis, substance-related disorders, and poorly controlled pain.

Management includes the treatment and elimination or correction of secondary causes, and may include a sleep assessment and polysomnographic examination if a primary sleep disorder is considered. Behavioral interventions to improve sleep hygiene and the elimination of psychoactive substances, such as caffeine, nicotine, and alcohol, should be initiated. If a major depressive episode is present, it should be treated as outlined in the discussion above. Judicious use of low doses of benzodiazepenes (e.g., oxazepam, lorazepam, clonazepam) is often useful, particularly if the sleep complaint is judged to be of an acute time-limited nature. Trazadone in low doses (50 to 150 mg PO qhs) is a very well tolerated and efficacious alternative, particularly if chronic use is anticipated. Patients taking trazadone need to be advised of the potential side effects of orthostatic hypotension and priapism and be aware of their emergency management.

PAIN

Pain is common in the course of HIV disease, affecting an estimated 60 percent of patients at some point in their illness course. Most patients experience more than one type of pain at any one time, and undermanaged pain can be a frequent cause of psychiatric morbidity. At the same time, pain may be amplified by coexistent and undiagnosed anxiety or depressive disorders. Pain is frequently undertreated, and there are many patient and health care provider barriers to adequate pain management. HIV-infected individuals who are female, less educated, or nonwhite, and those having a history of injection drug use have been shown to be consistently undertreated as pertains to pain relief. Pain may be related to HIV-associated conditions, including HIV neuropathy, headache, myopathy, arthritis, vasculitis, mucosal damage, organomegaly, tumors, and opportunistic infections. Pain may also be a consequence of medications used to treat HIV-related conditions, as in myopathy secondary to zidovudine, and neuropathy and pancreatitis secondary to ddI and ddC, or may be associated with chemotherapy, radiation or invasive procedures. Pain may also be related to other non-HIV-related conditions to which all patients are susceptible.

Pain management should focus on eliminating exacerbating factors and utilizing analgesics in a rational targeted manner. Pain severity should be determined by the patient and assessment should be made of whether the pain is persisting, worsening, or improving with management. A basic approach to analgesic use begins with the use of nonopioid analgesics with or without adjuvant medications and progresses through to the addition of weak opioids through strong opioids with attention to utilizing the strength and dosage necessary to achieve pain control. Regular pain medication to achieve baseline analgesia is preferred to as-needed dosing in order to eliminate serious exacerbations of pain that may be difficult to control.

Adjuvant pain medications include antidepressants, anticonvulsants, and topical analgesics. The HCAs amitriptyline and nortriptyline as well as the SSRI paroxetine have been shown to have strong analgesic properties, particularly for neuropathic pain, presumably by inhibition of paroxysmal discharges of damaged nerves. Full antidepressant dosages are often needed for analgesic effect, with a mean onset of analgesic effect seen beginning by day 3 of treatment and peaking at week 3. Paroxetine is the only SSRI to date that has been shown to have analgesic properties, though its effects are less than those of amitriptyline or nortriptyline. Antidepressants exert their analgesic effect independent of their antidepressant effect. Anticonvulsants, including valproic acid, clonazepam, and carbamazepine, may all be effective for neuropathic and hyperpathic pain syndromes. Topical analgesics like capsaicin may be quite effective for neuropathic pain in selected patients.

The management of pain in patients with histories of substance-related disorders is frequently problematic. Patients on methadone maintenance may require high doses of opioids to manage pain not only because of neuroadaptation from chronic methadone use but also because many HIV-related medications (e.g., rifabutin) may decrease methadone levels. Health care workers frequently become concerned about creating an addiction when using opioids, and attention is needed to judicious use with frequent monitoring of target symptoms, dosing schedules, and side effects. With difficult patients, a written contract discussed and agreed upon by both the patient and the care giver is a useful way to prevent future conflict over pain management. The contract can outline the target symptoms to be controlled, the medications to be used, the mode in which they will be dispensed, and provisions about repeat prescriptions. The open discussion of these issues helps to curtail negative feelings generated by perceived drug-seeking behavior and allows both parties to feel comfortable in pain management.

During terminal stages of HIV disease adequate pain relief is essential in the delivery of palliative care. High-dose opioids as well as antidepressants may cause delirium and confusion. The elimination of pain should be of highest priority. If another opioid cannot be substituted, low-dose haloperidol, 0.5 to 1 mg daily, may reduce the confusion, have mild analgesic effect, and allow adequate pain relief to be achieved.

CONCLUSION

HIV-infected individuals can experience a wide range of psychiatric morbidity related to both organic factors associated with CNS HIV infection and sequelae of advanced systemic disease, as well as the psychological and social factors that impact on the patient as they negotiate the challenges of the illness course. Most commonly, these factors intersect and require interventions directed at multiple levels. To intervene effectively, it is important to diagnose psychiatric and neuropsychiatric syndromes and implement appropriate targeted interventions. The following section will discuss psychotherapeutic interventions that can be used across diagnostic syndromes.

Suggested Readings

Brettle RP. HIV and harm reduction for injection drug users. AIDS 1991;5:125–36.

Coté TR, Biggar RJ, Dannenberg AL. Risk of suicide among persons with AIDS. JAMA 1992;268:2066–8.

Day JJ, Grant I, Atkinson JH, et al. Incidence of AIDS dementia in a two-year follow-up of AIDS and ARC patients on an initial phase II AZT placebo-controlled study: San Diego cohort. Neuropsychiatry Clin Neurosci 1992;4:15–20.

Fernandez F, Adams F, Levy JK, et al. Cognitive impairment due to

AIDS-related complex and its response to psychostimulants. Psychosomatics 1988;29:38–46.

Geleziunas R, Schipper HM, Wainberg MA. Pathogenesis and therapy of HIV-1 infection of the central nervous system. AIDS 1992;6:1411–26.

Halman MH, Worth JL, Sanders KM, et al. Anticonvulsant use in the treatment of manic syndromes in patients with HIV-1 Infection. J Neuropsychiatry Clin Neurosci 1993;5:430–4.

Hriso E, Kuhn T, Masdeu JC, Grundman M. Extrapyramidal symptoms due to dopamine-blocking agents in patients with AIDS encephalopathy. Am J Psychiatry 1991;148:1558–61.

Lipton, SA. Models of neuronal injury in AIDS: another role for the NMDA receptor? Trends Neurosci. 1992;15:75–9.

Maj M. Organic mental disorders in HIV-1 Infection. AIDS 1990;4:831–40.

Markowitz JC, Rabkin JG, Perry SW. Treating depression in HIV-positive patients. AIDS 1994;8:403–12.

Portegies P, Enting RH, de Gans J, et al. Presentation and course of AIDS dementia complex. AIDS 1993;7:669–75.

Sewell DD, Jeste DV, Atkinson JH, et al. HIV-associated psychosis: A study of 20 cases. Am J Psychiatry 1994;151:237–42.

Worth JL, Halman MH. HIV disease. In: Rundell JR, Wise MG (eds). APA Press Textbook of Consultation Liaison Psychiatry. Washington, DC: American Psychiatric Press (in press—publication 1996).

PSYCHOTHERAPY WITH HIV-INFECTED INDIVIDUALS

Mark H. Halman, M.D., F.R.C.P.C.

Psychotherapy is a treatment intervention, applied across a range of psychiatric disorders and emotional conditions, based primarily on verbal and nonverbal communication. Objectives of a psychotherapeutic process include symptom relief, crisis resolution, support during a period of stress, containment and processing of intense affects, resolution of long-standing intrapsychic conflicts, and characterologic change. There are several different types of psychotherapeutic models, ranging from classical psychoanalysis to supportive psychotherapy, each using different techniques to attain the specific goals of treatment. Central to all psychotherapeutic techniques is the establishment of a therapeutic relationship, the alliance through which the healing process occurs. The therapist must be able to listen in a meaningful fashion to the patient's conflicts, objectives, needs, strengths, and affects.

In general, psychoanalysis is the most intensive process,

aimed at resolution of long-standing conflicts and significant change of character structure. Psychoanalytically oriented psychodynamic psychotherapy is derived from psychoanalysis but is less intensive and more widely applicable. Both techniques attempt to achieve symptom relief and personality modification through the attainment of insight and the process of working through unconscious conflicts and motivations that frequently shape behavior. The therapist utilizes the techniques of active listening, empathy, questioning, clarification, confrontation, and interpretation to help the patient bring unconscious conflicts into conscious awareness, where they may be understood, accepted, and integrated. The timing and depth of interpretations will depend on the strength of the therapeutic alliance and the attunement of the therapist to the needs, anxieties, and defenses of the patient.

Supportive psychotherapy, by contrast, aims primarily for symptom relief with little emphasis on modification of personality or defensive structure. It is present based and attempts to mobilize existing defenses to reestablish the patient's level of functioning. In addition to active listening, it employs the techniques of reassurance, suggestion, education, and inspiration. The therapist aims to actively promote the therapeutic alliance and acts as a person with whom the patient can develop a consistent and stable caring relationship. In the context of this therapeutic relationship, affects can be contained and processed, crises can be faced and negotiated, and stability of function can be maintained. It is widely applicable and can be used short term and long term depending on the patient's needs.

Frequently there is movement between psychodynamic and supportive psychotherapies. During a crisis, a more supportive stance may be needed. With the resolution of a crisis and symptom relief, a patient may choose to explore the origins of the feelings roused during the crisis. Through insight and the working-through process, the patient may alter future responses to crises or be more prepared to handle the affects generated. The majority of HIV-infected patients referred for psychotherapy enter the process at a time of crisis, often with symptoms of depression or anxiety and a sense of being overwhelmed. Psychological defenses and coping mechanisms that had previously allowed for healthy and adaptation are no longer sufficient to cope with the cumulative stresses and psychological insults brought with HIV disease. The initial assessment period will aim to delineate the nature of the problem, the personality structure of the patient, and the objectives of treatment. Many patients will respond to a short course of supportive psychotherapy aimed at strengthening defenses and resolving precipitating crises. A smaller number will benefit from short- and long-term psychodynamic psychotherapy based on their therapeutic objectives, capacity for insight, motivation for change, and ability to enter into a trusting relationship where exploration of the intrapsychic world may be undertaken. Time is necessary to allow for trust to develop, to gain insight into the patient's life and view of themselves in the world, and to develop the therapeutic alliance necessary for the work to proceed. As the sessions unfold the assessment of the suitability of the therapeutic approach continues to ensure that treatment objectives are being met.

HIV disease can stimulate many psychological issues, beyond affects of anxiety, anger, and depression, that lead patients into psychotherapy. Different points along the disease spectrum may raise different issues to be processed. Isolation is a common theme expressed at many points, which psychotherapy may address and ease. A therapist may recognize the need for provision of information about HIV disease and be able to help the patient mobilize forces to access necessary community agencies and support groups. In other cases, the therapist may recognize long-standing conflicts that the patient has over issues of vulnerability and dependence or fears that are harbored over loss of control, against which the patient actively and unconsciously may defend. A psychodynamic exploration may help the patient recognize the need in earlier life for those defenses, provide an opportunity to work through the memories that continue to shape those defenses, and create a path toward insight into the present-day barriers and limitations that those defenses impose. A flexible stance and the capacity to listen objectively and empathically to the patient will guide the process to help diminish the isolation experienced.

Loss is another common theme that shapes many patients' experience. Loss may involve the loss of friends and partners through illness and death, the loss of material possessions and employment that is a frequent consequence of chronic illness, loss of supports as a consequence of stigmatization, and the loss of physical strength, capacity, and appearance that accompanies advancing illness. Central to the theme of loss is the mourning of lost hopes and dreams that a shortened life presents, often without having negotiated many of the life conflicts, tasks, and stages, such as intimacy and generativity, that help people who are preparing to die face their final life stage with integrity rather than despair. In communities that have been severely hit by HIV disease the experience of loss has become routine and commonplace. The psychological responses that follow from this can range from psychic numbing to unexplained anger or dysphoria to use of alcohol and drugs to soothe the feelings generated by repeated loss. Psychotherapy allows patients to talk about feelings generated by loss, validate the relationships that have been lost, and mourn lost experiences. Through talk, patients can release energies and affects that may otherwise be numbed or acted out in potentially self-harming manners. Psychotherapy allows patients to focus on interpersonal losses, grieve transitions and limitations imposed by illness, and aim to initiate change to adapt to their current life circumstances.

Some patients respond to the threat of impending illness with a desire to attain a greater degree of self-honesty and reflection and will enter psychotherapy at some point after seroconversion with the expressed intent of working through issues that have to that point been barriers to the formation of satisfactory intimate relationships. Others may aim to resolve feelings of shame and conflict over identity and sexual orientation or process issues that have impacted on self-esteem. Some patients will seek psychotherapy to deal with issues pertaining to their family of origin, partners, and friends. The anticipated role transition brought about by illness, the feeling of being a burden, and the fear of rejection are frequently discussed.

The indications for psychotherapy are by necessity as wide as the responses to the threats posed by HIV disease are highly varied. The challenge to the psychotherapist is to listen empathically and to delineate with the patient the goals of treatment. The skills of psychotherapists, their consistency, and their relative objectivity and neutrality establish a safe place for this process to occur, unencumbered by the rules that dictate friendships and family relations. Often patients simply wish to have a witness to their journey, someone who can validate their experience and help them to maintain a connection to the living world and affirm their continuation in the human condition. The psychotherapist will face many challenges in this work, including a need for flexibility in the framing of the therapy and powerful countertransferential issues frequently stimulated by a sense of helplessness against a powerful illness. Collegiality, supervision, consultation, and one's own safe place to process the emotions generated by the work are critical to continued satisfaction and availability to patients.

Suggested Readings

ARTICLES

Beckett A, Rutan SJ. Treating persons with ARC and AIDS in group psychotherapy. Int J Group Psychother 1990;40(1):19–29.

Hays RB, Turner H, Coates TJ. Social support, AIDS-related symptoms, and depression among gay men. J Consult Clin Psychol 1992;60:463–9.

Markowitz JC, Klerman GL, Perry SW. Interpersonal psychotherapy of depressed HIV-positive outpatients. Hosp Commun Psychiatry 1992;43:73–8.

Nichols SE. Psychosocial reactions of persons with the acquired immunodeficiency syndrome. Ann Intern Med 1985;103:765–7.

BOOKS

Cadwell SA, Burnham RA, Forstein M. Therapists on the Front Line: Psychotherapy with Gay Men in the Age of AIDS. Washington DC: American Psychiatric Press, 1994.

▬ PSYCHOTHERAPY WITH INDIVIDUALS SUFFERING FROM A DEVASTATING ILLNESS

Dalia Slonim, Psy.D., C.Psych.

PSYCHODYNAMIC PERSPECTIVE

A patient who is suffering from a devastating illness needs a place where both the dying process and death can be explored. Death is the only event concerning the whole psychobiological organism that is predictable beyond dispute once birth has taken place. As such, though almost never consciously, death became a developmental issue, and as such is best conceptualized within a developmental framework. It is difficult, perhaps impossible, to describe what psychodynamic approach, or what I prefer to refer to as the *deep psychotherapy approach* (Michael Eigen's term), is in the short space allotted to me here. The interested reader therefore will have to bear with me and seek additional resources if the interest is of size.

All of development—the construction of character, the ultimate form of individual psychopathology, mental health, and everything else human—is constructed out of the interaction between the inborn and unfolding givens of a person and the environmental inputs of his or her life. The inborn givens include the individual's capacities for bodily and object-related pleasures of various degrees of intensity, thought, perception, memory, internal signaling, and adaptation of all kinds. The environmental inputs include primarily the "whos" and the "hows" of the primary care takers. The whos refer to the presence of mother, father, extended family, and so forth and their ages and experiences in child rearing. The hows refer to the whole canopy of variables describing their behavior, reliability, and availability, their tension and ease, tendency to praise or blame, glow or share, forbid or entice, the models they provide for identification, and an endless list of others. In addition, the environmental input includes the adventitious events of an individual's life: illness, loss, physical attributes, degree of wealth, and on and on. The individuals who come to your office bring all of this and more with them. By way of example:

> Tom came to my office on a rainy day, on March 5, years ago; he was 28 years old, he had lost his partner 3 years prior, and he was found to be HIV-positive himself at that time. Looking back at my notes I notice that I wrote "neatly dressed and groomed young man—who reminded me of a magazine picture which advertises clothes, or other such items." As Tom looked so "together" I'm sure I started feeling somewhat self-conscious about my own appearance. This is not a small matter since appearance was indeed so important to Tom, and probably still is, though he is now too weak to act upon his need. Later, he would tell me that before coming to see me he'd change his clothes about three times and still feel that something was amiss. When he left my office that first time, and for nearly 6 months, I had a sense of total desperation, as if my whole being was spent, and the office was absolutely full of raw pain and anger. Anger which is born out of lost dreams and sheer terror. Tom revealed that he was "nothing" before his partner came to his life and he is "nothing" again since his partner died. He started feeling desperate at the age of 11 and at 15 made his first suicide attempt, with others to follow.

In my work with individuals who are battling HIV and its sequel AIDS, we often engage in a therapeutic process that deals with the tremendous pain these patients, mostly gay men, suffer throughout life, way before the virus enters their bodies. In light of the dying process, all the old losses resurface.

The meaning attached to loss, particularly loss of function—impairment deficit—which could occur as the result of illness, accident, or merely the life process itself, dates from early development, the period in which the professed significance of losses began to become firmly established. Most of the immediate effect of the loss of function—such as anxiety, deprivation and the strong need for restitution—stem from the fact that these conflicts are prevalent in childhood and continue throughout life to influence and govern some aspects of our behavior. Furthermore, the young child often equates the loss of function or certain functions with death. Hence an impairment of function has a causal relation to conflicts that center around loss and restitution and the relation of the loss of function to dying and death.

I cannot think of any other illness that is a better representation of an ongoing, acute, and unstoppable loss of function than those seen in AIDS, nor can I think of another group of people who are more sensitive to loss of function than my patients who suffer from this disease; this sense of loss of bodily function and control is anything but new to them. The experience of a child who finds himself or herself set apart from what is considered the world "goings on" is far different from that of a child who has not experienced this kind of alienation. It seems to me, without getting into the complex arena of how, why, and who is to be held responsible for what, that, in general, the patients I have seen who are ill with HIV have been experiencing loss from very early on in their lives, to the point where they often feel that the only answer could be to terminate life altogether so that this acute pain could come to an end. The form of loss I refer to here probably could be best described as a developmental loss, a loss that the child experiences in the process of growth and development—the breast, the bottle, being an only child. An endless procession of loss of gratifications that are experienced as secured, comfortable, and grounding. For the child who discovers that his or her attraction and desires are "different" from others, this discovery and its implications first and foremost superimposes on every other loss and at times tips the scale over to the unbearable. Later on, the discovery of the illness brings with it not only the very real, terrifying, and life-threatening current reality, but also a resurfacing of the old feelings that more often than not are left unresolved.

The task of the therapeutic process then becomes that of exploring the everyday occurrence of a very difficult physical reality together with an exploration of the emotional reactions to it *and* reflection over old issues that have become potent once again.

I often ask myself, can you take a patient further than you yourself have gone? I do not think you can. I do not mean by that, that a therapist would have to be infected with the same illness, suffer the same trauma, or sustain the same injury to be able to work with a patient. By way of example, if we examine the issue of sexuality, supposing that the therapist's own sexuality was never celebrated or acknowledged, how can he or she celebrate someone else's livelihood with them or help them discover their sexual self? The same is true for other parts of ourselves and in turn in our work trying to assist in the discovery of those parts in others. The issue of deterioration, death, and dying also falls into this category.

Paradoxically, though, through my work with patients suffering from a devastating illness I now travel to a place I've not yet been to. To beneficially work with patients who are dying, I had to ask myself: do I have the courage needed to accompany them to the edge of the cliff as far as we can go without actually falling off and look with them at the abyss below? While the "unthinkable anxieties," to quote W.D. Winnicott, become reality for the patient, the therapy has to always follow the two diverse, sometimes paradoxical lines: hope for and celebration of life as well as acknowledgment of the end and affirmation of the fears and trepidation that knowledge generates.

As mentioned, understanding of the stages of devastating illness rests on the concept of loss of function—deterioration in function is what we all experience as life goes on. In the context of a devastating illness, loss of function is, continues, ongoing and multifaceted. As one of my patients told me when we started talking about the dying process and his fear of it: "I don't want a messy death." Unfortunately, the consequence of this illness is most often what my patient referred to as "messy": disorder, depletion, deterioration, as well as intense and multiple losses. The issue then becomes coping with both losses and survival. Since as you go on fighting for your life you have to hand-in-hand mourn ongoing losses brought about by your survival: loss of the ability to work, loss of physical stamina, deterioration in appearance and, at times, in cognitive function.

Being a neuropsychologist, and familiar with what systemic illnesses do to one's thinking process, I can see the fluctuation in that ability in my patients who are suffering from AIDS. One patient said to me once, long ago, about a month before he died: "I don't seem to be able to think at all today, I just want to sit here and listen to the clock ticking away." A day later he was able to participate in a meeting and was quite able to follow discussion and suggested ways of handling difficult matters as they arose. This patient and others provide a good example of the fluctuating flavor of both cognitive ability and emotional state in patients with chronic and acute systemic illness. Nothing is stable or static in the body or in the psyche anymore. The psychotherapeutic treatment cannot remain oblivious to this reality, as it may become futile or, worse, destructive to the patient.

Often the patients who suffer from the disease carry with them a history of being misunderstood and experiencing the environment as alienated from them and as hostile toward them. For this reason, as well as others, the therapeutic contact needs to focus on the specific: the changing reality of every patient, at any given time.

Allow me to go back to my "top of the cliff" metaphor. What does standing on the cliff with your patient mean? It means just that. The essential therapeutic tools in the treatment of the dying patient are the therapist's availability as an object (by object, I mean a person, place, thing, idea, fantasy, or memory, invested with emotional energy—love or hate, or more modulated combinations of the two) and the therapist's reliability, empathy, and ability to respond appropriately to the patient's needs. One of the most important and beneficial points: always pay attention to the patient's needs and be as flexible as possible, since most everything else in the patient's life is out of his or her control and autonomy is highly restricted.

For me personally, an essential prerequisite of therapy with the devastatingly ill patient is consciously accepting my own countertransference (i.e., all of my own responses to the individual I work with). By the nature of the illness, this patient confronts us with an injury to our narcissism; the knowledge that things are getting worse and that the patient actually is dying inevitably mobilizes the therapist's childhood fears and anxieties and at the same time serves as a painful reminder of his or her own mortality. Defenses against either or both countertransferential reactions in large part explain why dying patients are often left to die alone and why positive thinking is so big in the treatment of the patient who is gravely ill. The therapist's own defenses and relative health distance him or her from the patient in one way or another and could interfere with his or her ability to respond to the patient's need. At times I feel that in some way it is a no-win situation, as any defense, be it denial, reassurance, repression, overprotectiveness, false optimism, or intellectualization, will interfere with my usefulness to the patient. My conscious awareness of the *sources* of these responses, as well as my ability to utilize and accept those feelings, almost always is therapeutic for the patient. Recently, in a workshop with people working as care givers, one member of the group asked me how not to be afraid of illness; my answer was, "how is it possible not to be afraid? I'm terrified myself."

Each and every one of my patients told me at one point or another that I do not understand their predicament. They are right, I don't fully grasp the enormity of their suffering or the intensity of their loss, and for now I remain on the edge of the cliff while they take one more step.

■ HIV TEAM APPROACH

Jane Sanders, R.N.

Ian Barton, M.S.W.

The diagnosis of AIDS presents a catastrophic episode in the life of an individual. The critical illnesses leading to inevitable mortality, which characterizes the course of this disease, further assault the sense of self of the client. It is the role of both hospital and community team members to support the client and his or her significant others through these vicissitudes. Links between hospital and community enable the client to marshall his or her resources through support, education, and advocacy no matter where he or she may be in the course of the illness.

A client's first AIDS-defining illness requiring hospitalization is often the first time the hospital HIV team meets the client and his or her supports. Also, it may be the time the client is first made aware that he or she is HIV positive and/or has AIDS. There are many emotional, psychological, and spiritual issues to be worked through. A care team composed of a varied number of health care professionals (i.e., nurse, physicians, social worker dietician, occupational therapist, physical therapist, chaplain, psychologist, pharmacist, etc.) will have multiple resources available to support the client and his or her family.

The team enables the client to maintain the essence of his or her true self in the face of adversity. This is achieved in several ways. The most important of these is continuous involvement of the client in decision making and planning of care and treatment. This means the client's wishes must be respected even if they are not in accordance with professional opinion of the time. The wishes surrounding disclosure of information, treatment choice, and counselling concerns must be respected even when the client is no longer able to speak for him or herself. Education and informed consent are examples of ways in which the team demonstrates respect for the integrity of the client, which empowers the client and his or her significant others to make the choices which best suit his or her needs.

The goal of the team is to enable the client to foster the perception of a "well self." The view of the self as "well" reduces the risk of the client falling into a "sick" role sooner than is necessary. In addition to the preservation of the personal self, the cultural context in which the client functions also defines his or her support network. Often there are a wide variety of cultural influences, ranging from ethnicity to differences in families of choice and families of origin.

The transition of self from "well" to "sick" involves many changes in the client's value system. Strongly held beliefs and value systems will be challenged greatly as the illness progresses. Respecting different choices at different times allows the client to be in control. This wellness stage generally involves a long period of time, often years. In the wellness stage the community provides the bulk of professional support. The hospital team has a greater role in the "sick" phase.

The client then enters this phase of chronic illness with periods of acute episodic crisis. With each episodic admission comes a gradual increasing awareness of mortality, which can result in feelings of fear, anxiety, powerlessness, and incidents of depression.

It is important that the client establishes strong rapport with a hospital primary care team member (e.g., a nurse) as it is through this linkage that there can be continuity of care through all hospitalizations. The client and his or her significant others can build a trusting relationship with this team member. This relationship fosters mutuality with the team member, client, and the significant others so that they can plan client-centered care together and their significant others are given opportunities to participate in the planning and execution of all care and are encouraged to join in care conferences. A multidisciplinary plan of care reflects a sensitivity to the client and significant others' expectations and goals.

Prior to discharge the appropriate community support should be identified by the primary care worker so that appropriate linkages can be made. As the client moves along the continuum, an increasing number of resources may have to be utilized. Early discharge planning with identification of community needs will facilitate a timely return home.

At this time the client may enter a phase where he or she addresses issues of wills, power of attorney, resuscitation, and living wills. Most clients will accept assistance facing these decisions. There will always be those who will reject all attempts to address these same issues. If they are judged competent to make that choice the decision must be respected. The health care professional must continue to support and encourage independence even as the basic needs of the client are increasing.

Deterioration in the client's medical condition that requires the cessation of work may have a considerable impact on his or her life situation. The client may face financial hardship, which requires dependence on government assistance. Existing housing may no longer be a viable option for the client and he or she may have to seek out other subsidized housing, which could lead to stigmatization. Individuals whose self-identity has been particularly linked to their jobs are further assaulted. They may struggle with decision making and feel increasingly out of control. Continuing debilitation, loss of self-esteem, and an increased awareness of impending mortality further challenge the client's ability to maintain equilibrium. The primary care nurse can facilitate a strengthened relationship with the significant others to support the client. The team may have to assist the family to decrease the interpersonal stresses on the client, particularly when his or her coping resources are being most actively challenged.

It is in the terminal stages of this illness that the benefits of a strong team support network are most evident. Sometimes the need for autonomy is so strong that it supersedes the issues of safety or health. It is critical that clients be encouraged to express wishes and input decisions to the last stages of their life. The team has a critical role in facilitating this decision making, although the wishes may be indicative of an ambivalence about living or dying on the part of the client. By remaining actively involved with the client and his or her supports through all the stages, the team provides a supportive and caring environment, which allows the client to proceed toward his or her death in the most humane manner possible.

■■■ SPIRITUALITY

The Rev. Peter Thompson, B.A., M.Div.

It should be abundantly clear that a diagnosis of HIV infection is much more than a "medical" or even a "health" crisis, for the patient's entire way of being in the world, or the relation to self and others, will be challenged and altered as the individual begins to live with HIV infection.

A simple blood test sets in motion profound changes in the lives of people who test positive for HIV. Many times the individual is completely asymptomatic and has been motivated to seek testing for any of a number of reasons, such as feared exposure, a change in intimate relationship, or even to qualify for insurance. Whatever the rationale for testing, its impact on the life of an individual and his or her intimates touches every aspect of their being. The stage is set for a crisis, a turning point in life. In fact, it is quite possible for a person to be in crisis with a diagnosis long before any serious physical manifestations begin to make themselves known. An HIV diagnosis is a spiritual crisis of major importance.

HIV-AIDS-RELATED CONSIDERATIONS

Experience of Rejection by Religious Institutions

- Some religious institutions have endorsed a view of the disease as punishment for immoral behavior.
- Early childhood attitudes and fears of a vengeful and condemning God frequently reemerge at times of crisis and may lay below a veneer of self-reliance and rejection of "religion."

- Many people with HIV/AIDS are from groups marginalized from mainstream society and experience associated guilt and shame.
- Others are stigmatized by the image of the disease (i.e., the "gay plague").

Distinction of Religion and Spirituality

While there is a close connection between the two, religion and spirituality are not synonymous. *Spirituality* is a dimension of human being, constitutive and integrative of being, transpersonal in essence but experienced in personal and immediate ways: making connections and meaning. *Religion* is an organized and politicized belief system, a product of reflection upon experience and tradition, having common beliefs (dogma) agreed upon by followers.

Use of Complementary Therapies

The search for wholeness and meaning has revived interest in ancient healing arts, many of which are spiritually based. These choices are frequently influenced and informed by an individual's spirituality, by beliefs about health and what affects it, by the notion of how the world around one can be influenced to ones advantage (one's *cosmology*).

Attitude toward Western Medicine

- The advent of HIV/AIDS has influenced individual expectations of medicine, making it less mechanistic and less curative, with more focus on quality-of-life issues.
- It has redefined the doctor–patient relationship and made it less prescriptive and more of a partnership.

These changes were shaped by underlying values and beliefs, ways of being in the world that enhance personal autonomy (i.e., adopting proactive, health-seeking behaviors as opposed to a passive victim stance).

Spirituality in Medical Settings

- There is a perceived conflict between science/medicine and spirituality.
- There is a belief that spirituality is rooted in a prescientific world view.
- There is much ancient wisdom and a growing body of

modern scientific data that sees a correlation between healing and spiritual energy.

Transpersonal Effects

Entire communities are affected by HIV, not only individuals. There is a spiritual energy emerging in the HIV/AIDS community: a movement from powerlessness, hopelessness, isolation and marginalization toward hope by seeking solidarity, and affirmation of personal identity, as well as compassion, openness, mutual self-help, and respect of the individual.

HIV/AIDS SPIRITUAL COMPLICATIONS

Persons dealing with HIV infection are challenged in their way of being in the world. Their understanding of who they are and how they relate to the world about them comes under a natural, if frequently painful, scrutiny. This examination reaches deeply into the realm of spirituality. It is in the dimension of spirituality that questions of relationship, meaning and purpose, being and not being, and ultimacy are struggled with and reflected upon. Some examples of the type of ultimate questions asked are: *Who am I? Why am I? Does my life matter?*

Emotions that include intense anger, rage, euphoria, loss, sadness, and despair have long ago been witnessed and enumerated by professionals working with HIV-infected individuals. What has frequently been missed is the close relationship between these emotions and the spiritual states that underlie them. Consequently, a dimension of care and healing has sometimes been neglected or avoided because of discomfort around spirituality on the part of the "patient" or/and "care giver." In fact, it is not unusual for care givers to miss expressions of spiritual distress by attending to the practical realities of a situation and not hearing the deeper concern of a person who expresses a desire to "go home" (concerns about dying) or feelings of "being alone" (concerns about abandonment) when surrounded by people busy taking care of physical needs.

There are many ways that an alert care giver may begin to gather information about a client's spirituality. Dreams and fears are important indicators of spiritual energy even when they may seem to have no basis in present reality or abilities. Regardless of whether one uses traditional or nontraditional ways to express and describe the energies of the spirit, these energies are dynamic, like the emotions. Like the emotions, they are neither good nor bad, but are simply expressive of human energy and spirit. It must be kept in mind that it is not outcomes that are paramount in the realm of exploring spirituality, rather, it is the recognition and sense of personal integration experienced by the client in the process that is of ultimate significance. The process of spiritual work may allow hope to arise in spite of physical disintegration, decline, and death. Spiritual work may help an individual move toward a sense of fullness, completion, and peace. Such movement on the spiritual level is life enhancing. Some positive indicators are as follows:

- **Political action:** linking with others so as to enhance one's connections, sense of power and meaning.
- **Self-care:** recognition of one's real needs and the resources to meet them.
- **Unconditional love:** self-acceptance, which includes knowledge of one's limits, a sense of completion and wholeness that transcends self.

Issues that may need to be worked through on a spiritual level include:

- **Loss:** Continuous life losses, of future plans and hopes, community, friends, income, status; erosion of personal identity, well-being, meaning.
- **Marginalization:** loss of self-esteem; may give rise to disenfranchised grief: *"Nobody knows my pain."*
- **Complicated grief:** repeated loss without adequate time to grieve or reintegrate: *"I am too numb to care anymore."*
- **Death:** questions and fears about the unknown; fears of retribution; fears about the process of dying, pain, and suffering; fears of loss of control, which may present as self-harming.
- **Hopelessness:** no purpose or meaning in life, past or present: *"There is no point."*
- **Judgment:** fears of rejection by friends, family, God; may present as self-rejection: *"Do I deserve this?" "I guess I got what I deserved."*
- **Survivor guilt:** having seen too many die; fears of being left behind: *"I don't deserve to be here";* sometimes presents as subtle self-destructive behavior.
- **Identity:** erosion of self concept: *"Who am I? Who will I become?"*

- *Abandonment:* feeling of being the sole survivor, feelings of worthlessness, that nobody cares: *"I can't let them know."*

CARE FOR THE CARE GIVER
The Rev. Peter Thompson, B.A., M.Div.

One of the most neglected aspects of HIV/AIDS care is the importance of self-care for the care giver, which can influence one's ability to provide ongoing empathic care. Many factors contribute to the unique stresses of those working as care givers in the field of HIV/AIDS. Some of these stresses are identified in what follows. This discussion is by no means exhaustive, nor are the stressors in order of priority. In fact, no such order exists, as stressors act in combinations, creating synergistic effects greater and more complex than if they operated in isolation.

STRESSORS RELATING TO HIV/AIDS CARE GIVERS

- *Age:* The HIV/AIDS population is generally young, sometimes younger than the care givers, thus triggering issues concerning the care giver's own fear of death.
- *Stigma:* Layers of stigma surround HIV/AIDS. In North America, the infected population has largely been from marginalized communities (i.e., gay men, IV drug users, and prostitutes). Some care givers believe these individuals are less deserving of care and thus continue the stigma. Care givers free of these prejudices frequently find that they themselves are stigmatized by family, friends, and coworkers who believe their efforts would be better spent on more deserving people.
- *Epidemic:* HIV/AIDS appeared in North America at a time when society was confident that disease could be controlled by medicine, and that major epidemics were a thing of the past. HIV/AIDS has reawakened deep-seated fears of disease and contagion, engendering attitudes that marginalize and stigmatize those infected.
- *Morbidity:* HIV-AIDS is fatal to all who contract it, and in the beginning of the epidemic, there were no effective treatments. The resulting death of hundreds of young

people has shaken prevalently held assumptions and beliefs about who dies, when we die, and why we die. The dominance of Western medicine and our beliefs about what constitutes healing began to fracture. This shift in perspective continues to have far-reaching consequences as care givers grapple with feelings of powerlessness and helplessness.

- *Fear of Contagion:* Education has been the key in helping care givers control their fears of working with those who carry an infectious fatal virus. However, these fears, as deeply seated as our creaturely fear of death itself, can recur in times of stress, such as when there has been an incident with contaminated body fluid. Education must be constantly reinforced, as care givers function daily amid persistent societal fears of HIV/AIDS.

- *Trauma:* Care givers are trained to repress their own needs and emotions in order to function in crisis. The care of people with HIV/AIDS involves continued exposure to emotionally demanding situations complicated by social, spiritual, medical, and political dilemmas. Such exposure diminishes natural recuperative powers and heightens the need for institutionally sponsored self-care programs, as does the attitude of many care givers that they should not use time and energy to meet their own needs.

CONTRIBUTORS TO STRESS/BURNOUT AS IDENTIFIED BY CARE GIVERS

- *Overload:* There is a large number of individuals to be cared for and many exhibit complex social, spiritual, medical, and political issues. At the same time the present context has engendered constant rethinking of relationships as we witness an on-going redefinition of beliefs about health and medical care.

- *Lack of Resources:* Care givers frequently experience an inability to provide adequate and necessary care despite their efforts to fill gaps in the system, often at their own time and expense.

- *Isolation:* Care givers may experience isolation when shunned by coworkers and friends due to their association with HIV/AIDS. The care giver's own HIV status may give rise to anxiety and further isolation.

- *Disenfranchised Grief:* Mourning is complicated by the issues of isolation and stigma as well as by the sheer volume of losses. Further complications in mourning may arise for the many care givers who are part of the communities most affected. Some care givers and/or their partners have HIV/AIDS, leading to stress in the workplace when deaths and personal losses occur that cannot be acknowledged.

- *Chaos:* Health care workers feel they are working in a war zone with no sense of order. The traditional relationships among care givers of different disciplines and between patients and care givers are in transition, and that which provided stability is lost.

- *Homo-/AIDS Phobia:* Care givers must cope with the fears and prejudices of coworkers. Alienated family members may reemerge during a health crisis and are sometimes in conflict with the patients' treatment decisions, personal beliefs, and expressed values. Care givers are frequently caught in complex dynamics around issues of confidentiality and decision making.

- *Structures:* Care givers experience frustration in providing continuity of care as a patient moves through a variety of settings. There is some overlapping of roles among care givers of different disciplines, and a variety of agencies as roles are redefined. Inability to effect change in institutional structures and policies, inappropriate supervision limiting the individual care giver's professional autonomy, and dealing with systemic problems by singling out individual care givers (i.e., scapegoating), are some of the most significant contributors to burnout named by care givers.

- *Roles:* Role definitions are in transition, corresponding to change in philosophies of health care and dealing with the projected, and frequently inappropriate, expectations of peers, superiors, patients, and families is a major contributor to stress and burnout.

STRATEGIES FOR CAREGIVERS

- *Memory Book:* Provision of a book wherein care givers may record and collect feelings, memories, stories, pictures, and poems that they associate with patients for whom they have cared. The contents of this book are confidential, and access limited to the professional and volunteer staff.

- *Peer Support Groups:* Many types of support groups are

successful, these include time-limited or on-going, open- or closed-membership, and specific topic or open-agenda groups. It has been noted that attendance is best for groups in which members are given paid time to attend.

- **Flex Time:** Flexibility in work hours, institutionally supported retreat days, and employer-scheduled mental health days on a regular basis help to ensure that care givers take adequate self care.

- **Debriefing Sessions:** An informal session following critical incidents, difficult deaths, or a series of deaths and case study reviews may help care givers identify problems but also can provide a place to vent feelings, recognize accomplishments, and strengthen team connections.

- **Memorial Gatherings:** Memorial gatherings provide a time apart for staff and volunteers to remember those for whom they have cared. The focus of this time is to allow care givers to find meaning in their own experiences. Staff should be allowed time to attend public memorial/funeral services if they so desire.

- **Memorial Funds:** Establishment of funds to be used at the discretion of staff for the needs of future patients helps staff have a sense of control in recognizing and meeting the comfort needs of clients.

- **Celebrations:** Events for staff and volunteers to recognize special days (i.e., major holidays, changes in team membership, recognition of special accomplishments) may help strengthen the sense of being a team and helps to normalize the mood of a unit or center.

- **Political Action:** Connecting with others around issues of common concern (e.g., walking in fundraisers such as "From All Walks of Life") and meeting together to strategize for change can empower individuals and overcome any sense of isolation and hopelessness.

- **Creative Therapies:** Free access for staff and volunteers to a variety of optional therapies that enhance personal growth and wholeness (e.g., art therapy, massage, Tai Chi, meditation) helps relieve stress and stimulate creativity and healthy emotional expression.

There is no perfect model for developing a program of care for care givers. Many of the observations described above are the distillation of detailed experiences of caregivers (presented in San Francisco at the 1992 "Care for the

Caregiver" Conference, sponsored by the Boston University School of Social Work).

What has emerged from many settings is a consensus that the need is great for institutionally sponsored care. Also, care givers have demonstrated considerable creativity in developing resources to suit their particular settings. Many care givers have found their own strength and hope emerging as they struggle together to find ways to meet their own needs in their own context.

Palliative Care and Pain Management

Mary Anne Huggins, M.D.C.M., C.C.F.P.

Dianna Drascic, B.Sc.N., M.Sc.N./A.C.N.P.

This chapter describes the role of palliative care medicine in the care of the patient with AIDS. First, the principles and practice of palliative care medicine are discussed, followed by the application of these principles to the care of the patient with AIDS.

The term *palliative care medicine* is used in the field of palliative care to emphasize the importance of the role of the physician and expert care in the management of patients with a terminal illness. Good palliative care implies good medical care with the involvement of expertise from the multidisciplinary team to provide active and agressive management of pain and other symptoms to improve the quality of life of the patient and help relieve suffering. Symptom control is of prime importance because without good symptom control in the physical sphere it will be difficult to deal with the multiple and complex issues that are also part of the palliative care of the patient. The members of the multidisciplinary team, including physicians, nurses, pharmacists, social workers, chaplains, dietitians, physical therapists, and occupational therapists, are experts in symptom control in the multiple areas of need in this patient population—physical, psychological, social, spiritual, functional, and legal/financial. Excellent assessment skills and coordination of services enhances the successful management of the terminally ill patient.

Thus, palliative care medicine

- Addresses pain and other physical symptoms.
- Addresses psychological, social, and spiritual issues.
- Is active, interdisciplinary care.

- Is directed toward relieving suffering and improving quality of life.
- Is not focused on curing or prolonging life.
- Can be a part of patient care at any stage of illness.

In the care of someone with AIDS, as in any terminal care situation, it is the meticulous attention to detail, the degree of good communication between all concerned, and the team work, with compassion, and understanding, which will make the ultimate difference to the quality of living and the dying, and the memories with which the patient's loved ones have to live on in the years to follow.

PRINCIPLES AND PRACTICE OF PALLIATIVE CARE MEDICINE

Palliative care can be delivered in a variety of ways and in a variety of settings. It can be delivered in the community to a patient at home, in a hospital on a dedicated unit, in a free-standing hospice, or as a consultation team service to patients being cared for by a speciality service. Palliative care can also be incorporated into the care delivered at outpatient specialty clinics or emergency wards as part of the patient's comprehensive medical management.

Palliative care is an approach to care that goes beyond the disease-focused, cure-oriented management to add patient-and-family-centered, problem-oriented care. The introduction of the palliative care team to the care of the patient has frequently occurred after attempts at treating the disease have been exhausted and the patient has been labelled "palliative," with an either/or view to the care. Alternatively and preferably, palliative care medicine should complement active, aggressive cure/disease-focused care and play a role from the stage of diagnosis onward. This role may increase in importance over time to become the total, final care of the patient.

- Death is acknowledged as a natural part of life.
- Physical symptoms, including pain, must be controlled (primary intent is to increase comfort and to reduce suffering).
- Other domains of symptoms/needs that need to be addressed:
  —psychological.
  —social and cultural.

—spiritual.
—financial.
—legal.
—functional.

- Patient and family are the unit of care (with *family* defined as any person close to the patient—in knowledge, concern, and affection).

- Care is person-centered, patient-directed.

- Care is delivered by a multidisciplinary team that coordinates and integrates activities of the care givers (physician, nurse, social worker, chaplain, lawyer, occupational therapist/physical therapist, dietitian, pharmacist).

- Care can be delivered at home, in hospital or hospice/palliative care unit—creation of a "home" wherever that may be.

- Respects the inherent worth, dignity and uniqueness of each person.

- Is guided by the ethics of autonomy, beneficence, nonmaleficence, justice, confidentiality, and truth-telling.

- Grief and bereavement support is supplied for family before and after death.

PALLIATIVE CARE MEDICINE FOR PATIENTS WITH AIDS

AIDS challenges palliative care providers to apply the principles of palliative care in a situation that stretches and tests the limits of palliative care. Palliative care, as in the hospice/palliative care movement, was initially conceived for the care of the terminally ill cancer patient when the disease treatment could no longer achieve a cure. The palliative care of the person living with AIDS shares many elements of the care of the patient in the terminal phase of cancer but also has some significant differences. These differences are due partly to the pathophysiology of AIDS and its epidemiology. The natural history of AIDS is still evolving and disease patterns have changed over the past decade, partly as a result of the impact of treatment of HIV infection and the progress in the prevention and management of the opportunistic infections. People are living longer but may end up with a heavier, multisystem disease burden. In the advanced/terminal phase AIDS can present complex and challenging problems.

Common features of AIDS that differ from those of most terminally ill cancer patients include the following:

- Younger age group.

- Multisystem disease, which may result in (often concurrently)
  —Blindness.
  —Paralysis.
  —Neuropathy.
  —Confusion.
  —Myopathy.
  —Skin disorder.
  —Severe diarrhea.
  —Intractable nausea.

- Misery due to many coexisting physical problems.

- Large number of drugs, vitamins, and supplements being taken for years, some experimental and many overwhelmingly expensive.

- Difficulty in identifying the terminal phase of the disease—very sick patients may improve and opt for acute treatments.

- Treatments such as blood transfusions, total parenteral nutrition and IV therapies are often given to maintain quality of life in the terminal care AIDS patients.

- Lengthy dying process—patient may be unconscious for a week or more.

- Most people with AIDS know more about their disease and its treatment than the people caring for them and demand involvement in their care and treatment.

- Fear, prejudice, and lack of compassion for AIDS patients are evident in many segments of society.

- Social isolation of patients and their families.

- Homelessness or inadequate housing.

- Need for long-term supervisory care and housing for disabled people.

- Need for determination of guardians for children whose primary care giver(s), usually the mother, is dying and who may be dying themselves.

- Complexity of assessing capacity and competency due to neurologic impairments—important to address power of attorney for personal care and financial affairs early in the course of the illness.

- Prevalence of HIV among disenfranchised populations, especially the poor, homeless, and substance abusers.*

The Disease Trajectory of AIDS

The disease trajectory that seems to characterize AIDS over time has been described as a "roller-coaster," with the patient's status dramatically changing up and down over time as life-threatening illnesses are treated. The disease trajectory of AIDS or the stages of AIDS can be classified as

Early→ Progressive→ Advanced→ Terminal

This distinction attempts to help determine the focus of treatment but the transitions are gray and the time at which the term *terminal* is used is partly determined by the disease burden and partly by the person carrying that burden. Control and autonomy in decision making around treatment are very important issues for a person with AIDS. It is vital to recognize not only where the disease "is at" but also where the patient stands and begin there with the decision-making process. The goals of any treatment must also be clear and agreed upon, and these goals may vary over time and from symptom to symptom.

The major focus of palliative care medicine is symptom control. In AIDS, the symptoms of the disease (immune deficiency) are the opportunistic infections (OI) and cancers as well as the direct effects of HIV infection. The chief symptoms that patients complain of are frequently related to the OI and cancers. Prevention of OI and treatment of specific OI and cancers that result from the immune deficiency is symptom control, but it is also part of the aggressive disease-control focus on investigations and treatments that aim to prolong life. Prevention and treatment of OI is actually "palliative care medicine" as treatment is not directed at the underlying disease process (immune deficiency). Thus palliative care for those living with AIDS can be more narrowly defined as care in the far-advanced/terminal phase when aggressive investigation is abandoned, but it is recognized that the principles of palliative care apply throughout the course of the illness. In the terminal phase treatment focuses on symptoms that the patient complains about regardless of cause and disease-specific treatment is

---

Adapted from Sims R, and Moss V. Terminal care for people with AIDS, 2nd ed. London: Edward Arnold Publishers, 1994, reprinted by permission.

limited to those strategies that contribute to symptom management or can be expected to contribute to quality of life and, only secondarily, to quantity of life.

Exactly when this transition takes place varies from patient to patient and from symptom to symptom within the same patient. Some patients may choose to continue aggressive therapy against cytomegalovirus (CMV) to prevent blindness but elect not to investigate or treat aggressively any pneumonia and to treat presumed *Pneumocystis carinii* pneumonia only with oral medication. This may be based on a desire for greater quality of life (preserve vision) over quantity of life (cure pneumonia).

End-of-Life Decision Making, Including "Do Not Resuscitate" Directives

Many important and difficult areas must be resolved to ensure patient-centered and -directed care as well as to meet the needs of the family. These include an advanced directive in some form (written, oral, taped), a will, establishment of powers of attorney for both personal and financial affairs and confirmation of child care arrangements both pre- and postdeath. Important considerations in this process are the wishes of the patient and/or his or her appointed decision maker. It is thus imperative to know the patient's wishes and desires for care and be clear with the patient about the intent of treatment. The intent of treatment is crucial in determining the appropriateness of any proposed treatment, including cardiopulmonary resuscitation (CPR). CPR is a treatment like any other and should not be offered when it is not a viable option. In end-stage multisystem failure the chances of meaningful survival postresuscitation are minimal. Any discussions regarding resuscitation and "Do not resuscitate" (DNR) orders must be handled with great care and sensitivity to the person's overwhelming vulnerability. The discussions must involve explanations of what can and will be done to provide for their comfort, care, and dignity at all times. Often, an overt discussion regarding DNR issues is not necessary once the patient's wishes regarding goals of care are known. The decision not to be resuscitated is often part of the decision to forego aggressive investigation and treatment and may mark the transition to the terminal phase. The patient and or family must never be led to feel that they are solely responsible for life and death decision making. It is the responsibility of the care provider to review viable options and goals of treatment with the patient and family and help them to determine a satisfactory strategy. It is also important to have the decision-making process in place while the patient is able to express his or her wishes and to have a designated decision maker/medical power of attorney appointed by the patient for the time when he or she may become unable to express his or her wishes. Palliative care needs to be patient-directed care, with a partnership between patient and care giver. It is also clear that the coordination and integration of care between primary care giver, specialty care giver, and the palliative care giver is crucial to the successful, total care of the person living with AIDS throughout the disease trajectory.

Palliative Needs Identified for Patients with AIDS

- Physical symptom control/management.
- Psychological support.
- Interpersonal support.
- Bereavement support.
- Independent living.
- Legal/financial support.
- Lifestyle/cultural/ethnic/considerations.
- Spiritual support
- Women's issues of childbearing, contraception, family, guilt about passing it on to her children, caring for ill and dying children while she is dying.
- Service delivery.

The palliative care needs of AIDS patients as outlined above may seem overwhelming. As physicians try to deal with the pain and other physical symptom control needs, they also need to be aware of the whole gamut of other issues affecting the patient and the family and their effect on the patient's experience of physical symptoms. This emphasizes the need for multidisciplinary team approach to the terminally ill patient. The physician is one member of a multidisciplinary team who are skilled and have a range of expertise to meet the patient's needs as outlined above. Even if all these needs cannot be met at one specific time, it is important to evaluate the multiple needs of the patient and try to coordinate with the other team members to formulate a plan to address the other concerns.

APPROACH TO SYMPTOM MANAGEMENT IN THE CARE OF PERSONS WITH AIDS

Common symptoms in terminal AIDS*:

- Pain   %

Neuropathic	22
Pressure sore	12
Visceral (chest/abdominal)	10
"Total body"	9
Headache	8
Joint	7
Epigastric/retrosternal	7
Myopathic	5
Anorectal	4

- Other common symptoms

General debility/weight loss	61
Anorexia	41
Confusion/dementia	29
Nausea/vomiting	21
Depression	20
Skin problems	
Dry skin	19
Seborrheic dermatitis	14
Scabies	7
Molluscum contagiosum	4
Psoriasis	1
Cough	19
Diarrhea	18
Constipation	18
Dyspnea	11
Paralysis	8
Patients admitted moribund	8

In all stages of management of a patient with AIDS it is important to make an accurate diagnosis of the cause of a symptom in order to determine whether or not it is possible to treat the underlying cause for symptom relief. The differential diagnosis is based initially on the history and the physical examination weighed in the context of the possible cause of that symptom in AIDS. If the cause of the symptom is not clear from history and physical examination alone, the decision whether or not to pursue aggressive diagnostic

*Based on 100 patients admitted to a hospice, in order of frequency. Sims R, and Moss V. Terminal care for people with AIDS, 2nd ed. London: Edward Arnold Publishers, 1994, reprinted by permission.

evaluation should be based on the likelihood of finding a treatable cause, the stage of the illness, concurrent medical problems, the harm:benefit ratio of each test and, most importantly, the wishes of the informed patient.

Treatment decisions follow the same format. Knowledge of the treatment options for the underlying cause of a symptom forms the basis for decision making. Once again, the stage of the illness, the harm:benefit ratio of treatment, and the wishes of the patient determine treatment decisions.

Symptom management should include the following:

1. Determine the cause of symptoms—empirically or based on investigation.

2. Treat the cause if possible and appropriate.

3. Treat the symptom itself.

The chief goal in caring for AIDS patients in the last stages of life is to maximize comfort, function, and autonomy in the face of progressive physical deterioration.

MANAGEMENT OF COMMON SYMPTOMS IN ADVANCED/TERMINAL AIDS

Pain

Pain is a common symptom in advanced AIDS. As with all symptoms, it is important to determine the cause of the pain and treat the underlying cause if possible. The symptom of pain should be managed in conjunction with any treatment aimed at the cause.

In a prospective study of 100 consecutive patients admitted to a hospice program, significant pain whose underlying cause was not directly treatable was present in 53 patients, with 64 pain problems. The type of pain was*:

	No. (%)
Peripheral neuropathy	19 (34)
Abdominal pain	12 (23)
Headache	10 (19)
Skin pain	9 (17)
Oropharyngeal pain	4 (8)
Chest pain	3 (6)
Diffuse aches	2 (4)
Unrelated to AIDS	5 (9)

---

*Schofferman, J. Pain: Diagnosis and management in the palliative care of AIDS. J Palliat Care 1988;4(4):46-49. Reprinted by permission.

The causes of pain in AIDS include the following:

- Pain related to HIV/AIDS
  —HIV neuropathy
  —HIV myelopathy
  —Kaposi's sarcoma (KS)
  —Secondary infection
  —Organomegaly
  —Arthritis
  —Vasculitis
  —Myopathy/myositis

- Pain related to treatment of HIV/AIDS
  —Antiretrovirals
  —Antivirals
  —PCP prophylaxis
  —Antituberculosis drugs
  —Chemotherapy (vincristine)
  —Radiation therapy
  —Surgery
  —Procedures

- Pain in women with HIV/AIDS
  —Pelvic pain syndrome
  —Gynecologic malignancies
  —Gynecologic infections

- Pain unrelated to HIV/AIDS

The approach to pain in the person with AIDS is similar to that of a person with cancer. A pain assessment is important to determine the site, quality, mode of onset, intensity, aggravating and alleviating factors, and associated symptoms. The WHO cancer pain management strategy can be used, which involves a stepwise approach to pain management that depends on the severity of the pain (Fig. 10–1).

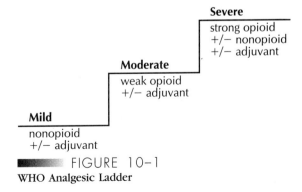

FIGURE 10–1
WHO Analgesic Ladder

This approach to pain management has been validated in the management of pain in the cancer patient and a study in ongoing to validate this approach in AIDS patients.

Nonopioids

Acetylsalicylic acid (ASA)	650 mg q4h for fever or pain 975 mg q6h for inflammation
Acetaminophen and other nonsteroidal anti-inflammatory drugs (NSAIDs)	650–1000 mg q4h

Weak opioids

Codeine	30–120 mg PO q4h
Oxycodone	10–15 mg PO q4h

Strong opioids

Morphine	Start at 10 mg PO q4h, titrate dose to pain; SC/IV dose is 1/2 PO dose
Hydromorphone	Start at 2 mg PO q4h, titrate dose to pain; SC/IV dose 1/2 PO dose Hydromorphone:morphine dose 1:5 ratio

Adjuvants

Steroid—dexamethasone	4 mg PO BID–QID
Antidepressants—amitriptyline	25–150 mg PO qhs
Anticonvulsants	
carbamazepine	100–200 mg PO BID, max 400 mg PO TID
valproic acid	250–500 mg PO qhs, max 1000–1500 mg PO qhs
Membrane stabilizers	
mexilitine	50–100 mg PO BID, max 400 mg PO daily

For treatment of mild to moderate pain start with a peripherally acting analgesic such as acetaminophen or a nonsteroidal anti-inflammatory agent such as ASA or ibuprofen *on a regular basis and not PRN*. If the pain is not adequately controlled, add a weak opioid such as codeine or oxycodone. These are often used in combination with ASA or acetaminophen and their dose is limited by that component. Codeine has a ceiling of analgesia at approximately 180 mg PO. If the pain is not well controlled or is severe a strong opioid should be used, such as morphine or hydromorphone. They are both strong opioid agonists with a 5:1 potency ratio and no ceiling to their analgesic effects. They have a similar spectrum of side effects and toxic effects but in the same patient these may differ, allowing a switch if side effects of one become too difficult to manage. All opioids cause constipation and preventive treatment should be started, usually with a stool softener and a stimulant (docusate and senna glycosides). In the AIDS patient, diarrhea may already be a problem and may benefit from the constipating effects. Nausea is a frequent side effect, especially in the first few days of treatment and in the patient who is already experiencing nausea, haloperidol 0.5 to 1.0 mg PO/SC TID or even 2 mg PO/SC qhs can be helpful, as can prochlor-perazine 5 to 10 mg PO/PR q4h.

The strong opioids must be given on a regular schedule, usually q4h around the clock. It is important to add a rescue or breakthrough dose, usually at one half the q4h dose for pain that occurs before the next scheduled dose. If the pain regularly appears before the next dose is due, the q4h dose needs to be increased. The oral route for administration is preferred but opioids may also be given IV, SC, buccally, and rectally. Because the elixir preparation may be absorbed buccally, the analgesic can be continued even in the moribund patient with small volumes of the concentrated liquid. Injections can usually be avoided but could be given SC through a butterfly needle left in place.

Once a dose of morphine that controls the pain is established, one could switch to the sustained release formulation for convenience. This may work well when the pain is stable. With pain that is increasing or difficult to control, the immediate-release tablets or liquid provide greater flexibility and control of dosing.

The initial dose of morphine or hydromorphone depends on the severity of the pain and the patient's previous opioid exposure. The dose may be increased to control the pain, and doses will need to increase as the amount of pain increases. There is no upper limit to opioid dosing. Doses depend on how much drug is needed to control each particular pain.

Many patients and physicians are hesitant or reluctant to use the strong opioids because of the myths surrounding them. Patients have concerns about the "meaning" of being on morphine, think that the drugs are only used at the "end," and wonder if starting morphine means their end is near. They also fear starting "too early" and try to wait until they "really need it" for fear of running out of effective analgesia at the end. Both patients and care givers have fears about the issue of addiction to the opioids, and this is an important barrier to effective pain control in terminal illness.

Morphine can be used at any point in an illness when the severity of the pain requires a strong analgesic. There is no ceiling to the analgesic dose, so as the severity of the pain increases, increasing doses of morphine will offer increased pain control. Opioid analgesics when used appropriately for the control of pain do not lead to addiction and should not be withheld when needed. *Psychological dependence* or *addiction* is used to mean a pattern of drug use characterized by a continued craving for an opioid which is manifest as compulsive drug-seeking behavior leading to an overwhelming involvement with the use and procurement of the drug. Patients controlled on morphine for pain do not exhibit drug-seeking behaviors. Dosing is usually stable while the pain level is stable and increasing need usually implies increasing pain. When the pain levels decline, the dose of the opioid may be decreased. There may be physical dependence when on high doses for a period of time and the medication may need to be tapered. This physical dependence is not addiction.

Not all types of pain are opioid responsive. Certain specific pains benefit from the addition of adjuvant medication (coanalgesic) or other nonpharmacologic interventions. The adjuvants are usually used in conjunction with an opioid and can change an opioid nonresponsive pain into a opioid responsive or partially responsive pain.

Adjuvants for Some Pain Syndromes

Bone pain or inflammation	NSAIDs, ASA
Raised intracranial pressure	Dexamethasone
Neuropathic pain	
Nerve pressure pain	Dexamethasone
Nerve destruction	Antidepressants
Deafferentation	Anticonvulsants
Neuralgia pain	Anticonvulsants
Gastritis/ulcer	Prokinetic agent
	H_2 blocker
	Cytoprotective agent
Rectal/bladder spasms	Chlorpromazine
	Anticholinergic drugs
	Opium + belladonna supplements
Muscle spasm pains	Diazepam, clonazepine
	Baclofen

Use of Complementary Therapies as Nonpharmacologic Adjuvants to Symptom Management

As research into the management of pain and other symptoms by complementary therapies continues, several therapies are becoming increasingly accepted by care providers and patients, including massage, acupuncture, acupressure, body-energy work, relaxation, visualization, imagery, music and art therapy, naturopathy, and herbs. Therapies should be provided by experts sensitive to the complexity of needs experienced by this population.

Pain Syndromes in AIDS

NEUROPATHIC PAIN.   Peripheral neuropathy may be due to direct involvement of nerves with HIV or CMV, chemotherapy, antiretrovirals, or an associated medical or metabolic problem. This neuropathy is more common in the feet and legs than in the upper extremity. The pain is an unpleasant burning or tingling pain that is made worse with walking and standing. There is often an aching component. Sensory examination may show decreased sensation or hyperesthesia, or be normal. There may or may not be impairment of motor function with loss of deep tendon reflexes. This pain is often difficult to control. It is managed with a combination of an opioid and a tricyclic antidepressant such as amitriptyline 10 to 50 mg PO, given at night as it can be sedating. NSAIDs can also be added. If the antidepressants are not helpful, anticonvulsants or mexilitine could be tried.

Topical capsaicin ointment 0.025 to 0.075% has been used with ambiguous results, although it has some success in diabetic peripheral neuropathy. Nonpharmacologic methods such as transepidural nerve stimulation or acupuncture may also be tried.

MUSCULOSKELETAL PAIN.   Joint pains and myalgias may be related to the rheumatologic manifestations of HIV, HIV or zidovudine myositis, muscle inflammation, or general debility and muscle wasting.

These pains can be responsive to acetaminophen, NSAIDs, and opioids, often in combination, or with strong opioids alone. NSAIDs are useful when there is an inflammatory component.

ABDOMINAL PAIN.   The causes of abdominal pain include the following:

- Retroperitoneal adenopathy due to infection or malignancy.

- Intra-abdominal lymphoma.
- Ascites.
- Intestinal lymphoma.
- Kaposi's sarcoma.
- Hepatosplenomegaly
  —Viral.
  —Lymphoma.
  —*Mycobacterium avium* complex
- Cholangitis.
- Diarrhea/constipation.

Determining the cause of abdominal pain can help in directing management. Visceral pain, such as the pain from an enlarged liver, often responds to strong opioids. When tumor is involved, decreasing peritumor edema with steroids can reduce the pain.

HEADACHE. The causes of headache include the following:

- Direct involvement of the brain (HIV encephalopathy).
- Intracranial masses
  —Toxoplasmosis.
  —Lymphoma.
- Meningitis.
- Cryptococcus.
- Non-HIV-related
  —Vascular, migraine.
  —Tension.
  —Medication.

Again, the approach involves treating the underlying cause if appropriate and possible. If the pathophysiology involves raised intracranial pressure, dexamethasone may be useful. Acetaminophen, NSAIDs, and opioids are used in the stepwise protocol as outlined above. Use of nonpharmacologic modalities, such as relaxation and massage, is also important.

EPIGASTRIC PAIN. The causes of epigastric pain include the following:

- Esophagus
  —Candidiasis.
  —Herpes.
  —CMV.
  —Lymphoma.

—Treatment (radiation therapy).
—Reflux.

■ Stomach
  —Gastritis.
  —Peptic ulcer disease.
  —Gastric stasis.

If it is appropriate, treat the cause with antifungals, antivirals, antiulcer therapy, antacids, or prokinetic agents. The mucosal protective agent sucralfate may help. Opioid analgesics are often necessary in addition to other measures. Viscous lidocaine can help as a local anesthetic but must be used cautiously.

OROPHARYNGEAL PAIN.   Causes of oropharyngeal pain include the following:

■ Candidiasis (common).

■ Herpes simplex.

■ Kaposi's sarcoma.

■ Carcinoma.

Candidiasis should be treated aggressively with both oral and topical antifungal therapy. Good oral hygiene is important and there are a variety of mouthwash solutions available. A simple solution of salt and sodium bicarbonate can be useful to gargle and swish and spit frequently. Other components can include viscous lidocaine, peroxide, and Kaopectate.

SKIN PAIN.   The causes of skin pain include the following:

■ Pressure sores.

■ Kaposi's sarcoma.

■ Herpes simplex lesions.

■ Herpes zoster lesions.

■ Post herpetic neuralgia.

Pressure sores need aggressive skin care once they occur. More importantly, should be prevented with measures such as egg-crate mattresses, frequent turning, and skin protection from urine and feces. Once they occur they should be treated aggressively. Viral lesions may need acyclovir orally and topically. Pain management is approached in the usual stepwise fashion. Postherpetic neuralgia may benefit from carbamazepine or amitriptyline for neuropathic pain.

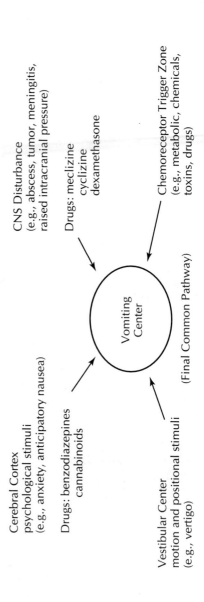

CNS Disturbance
(e.g., abscess, tumor, meningitis,
raised intracranial pressure)

Drugs: meclizine
cyclizine
dexamethasone

Chemoreceptor Trigger Zone
(e.g., metabolic, chemicals,
toxins, drugs)

Cerebral Cortex
psychological stimuli
(e.g., anxiety, anticipatory nausea)

Drugs: benzodiazepines
cannabinoids

Vomiting
Center

(Final Common Pathway)

Vestibular Center
motion and positional stimuli
(e.g., vertigo)

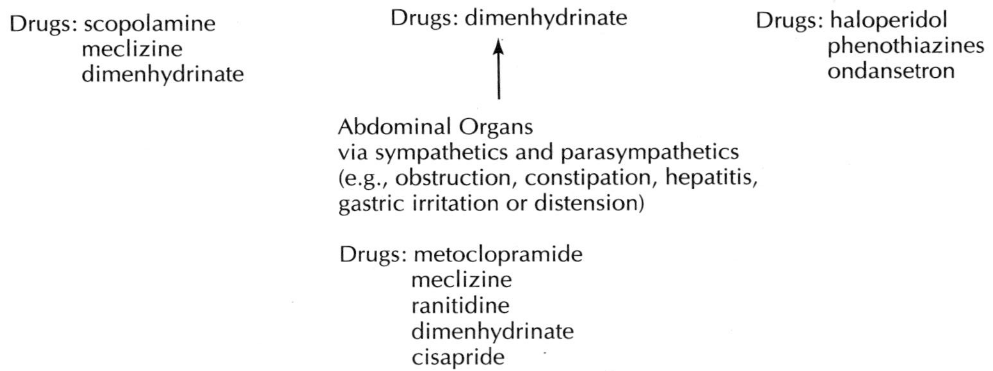

Drugs: scopolamine
meclizine
dimenhydrinate

Drugs: dimenhydrinate

Drugs: haloperidol
phenothiazines
ondansetron

Abdominal Organs
via sympathetics and parasympathetics
(e.g., obstruction, constipation, hepatitis,
gastric irritation or distension)

Drugs: metoclopramide
meclizine
ranitidine
dimenhydrinate
cisapride

FIGURE 10–2
Pathophysiologic Mechanisms of Nausea

Nausea

Nausea as a symptom is very common and is often difficult to manage. Nausea can be caused by a variety of pathophysiologic mechanisms, with a final common pathway involving the vomiting center in the medulla oblongata (Fig. 10–2). The different possible etiologies of the complaint of nausea require different choices of antiemetics for their management.

Common drugs in the treatment of nausea include the following:

Dimenhydrinate	50 mg PO/IV/IM/PR q6h
Prochlorperazine	5–20 mg PO/IM/IV/PR q6h
Metoclopramide	10–20 mg PO/IV QID
Haloperidol	0.5–5 mg PO/IM/SC/IV q8h
Scopolamine	0.4 mg PO/SC q8h
Cyclizine	50 mg PO/IV/SC q8h
Meclizine	25–50 mg PO q8–12h
Methotrimeprazine	25–100 mg PO/SC/IM q8–12h
Chlorpromazine	25–100 mg PO/IM/PR

Different antiemetics with different mechanisms of action may be used in combination to control nausea. These medications often have unwanted extrapyramidal side effects and benztropine may be necessary to treat this.

The approach to management of nausea is to determine its possible causes and choose an antiemetic or combination of antiemetics based on the possible causes.

Respiratory Symptoms

Cough and dyspnea are common symptoms and are often associated or feared to be associated with ominous causes. There are a number of causes, including infection, Kaposi's sarcoma involvement in the lung, or pneumonitis, some of which are treatable. The exact diagnosis may not be determined and therapy is often empiric. It is often the decision of whether or not to treat a pneumonia that marks the shift to terminal care. Many patients want to attempt to treat pneumonia and oral antibiotics are often used, with IV antibiotics thought to be too aggressive. It is important to discuss with the patient what the goals of treatment are.

Management of cough includes the use of suppressants:

Codeine	30–60 mg PO q4h
Hydrocodone	5–15 mg PO q4h
Morphine	5–10+ mg PO/SC q4h

Bronchodilator (salbutamol)	2.5–5 mg q4h
Humidity	
Soothing syrup (cough syrup, honey)	
Steroid (dexamethasone)	2–4 mg PO

Management of SOB/dyspnea includes:

Morphine	5–10 mg PO/SC/IV q4h or increase of 50 percent of usual dose
Benzodiazepine (diazepam)	5–10 mg PO/IV and 5–20 mg qhs
O_2	
Diuretic for pulmonary edema (furosemide)	20–40 mg PO/IV
Dexamethasone for lung KS	4 mg PO BID–QID
Bronchodilator (salbutamol)	2.5–5 mg q4h
Positioning	

Diarrhea

The causes of diarrhea include:

- Cryptosporidium—treat with paromomycin (Humatin).
- Lactose intolerance.
- Other infections.

The underlying cause should be treated if possible.
To control diarrhea:

- Loperamide (Imodium) 2–4 mg BID–QID.
- Diphenoxylate HCl (Lomotil) 5 mg TID–QID.
- Opioids—dose titrated to response.

Dementia/Neuropsychological Symptoms

Dementia and other neuropsychological symptoms are difficult for the patient, family, and care givers to manage. The goal of treatment should be to provide a comfortable, alert, safe, and manageable patient.
Symptoms can include:

- Mood and behavioral changes.
- Restlessness.
- Agitation.
- Anxiety.

- Emotional lability.
- Paranoia.
- Psychosis.
- Insomnia.

  Treatment options include

- Behavioral modification.
- Environmental modification.
- Medication.

  Drugs commonly used include

Haloperidol	1.5–5 mg PO/IM/SC daily (HS helpful)
Loxepine	10–25 mg PO/IM BID–TID
Lorazepam	0.5–2 mg PO/SL q4–6h

Patients with AIDS are very sensitive to psychotropic medications, including their side effects. Benztropine 2 mg PO/SC daily–BID is often necessary for the extrapyramidal side effects.

Anorexia and Wasting

The symptoms of anorexia and wasting can be a direct effect of HIV infection and difficult to reverse. Total parenteral nutrition has been attempted to improve the nutritional status of patients but its value has not been proven. Medications that may be helpful include

- Megestrol 40–80 mg PO BID–QID.
- Periactin 4 mg BID–QID.
- Dexamethasone 2–4 mg PO BID

Nutritional counseling may also be effective.

Other Needs

Psychological/Emotional Needs

- Need to maintain hope.
- Need for honesty.
- Need to raise painful and difficult issues.
- Need to overcome feelings of isolation.
- Need for encouragement and motivation.
- Need to be valued and be of value.
- Need for care giver's time.

Symptoms and issues include

- Anger.
- Guilt.
- Loss.
- Grief.
- Fear.
- Loss of control.
- Loss of body image.
- Depression (loss of a future).

Interpersonal Support

- Relationships.
- Social isolation.
- Discrimination.

Bereavement Support

- Family.
- Partner.
- Multiple losses.

Independent Living

- Care at home.
- Respite care.
- Transportation.
- Special accommodation.
- Day care.
- Income sources.

Legal/Financial Support

- Patients' rights.
- Informed consent.
- Will.

Lifestyle

- Gay lifestyle.
- Homophobia.
- IV drug use.

Cultural/Ethnic

- Funeral.

Spiritual

- Death concerns.
- Existential concerns
  —Value.
  —Meaning.
- Afterlife.
- Past religious teaching.

Service Delivery

- Facilities.
- Staff.
- Home care.

These issues also need to be addressed at all stages of the disease. This is best done with a multidisciplinary team, as no one person can expect to try to meet the variety of needs alone. It is important to involve nurses, social workers, chaplains, occupational therapists, physical therapists, pharmacists, nutritionists, and community agencies in the care of the patient in a coordinated and consultative manner.

PALLIATIVE CARE FOR WOMEN WITH HIV DISEASE

Women with HIV disease present a particular set of issues, distinct from the care of the male population with similar disease. Women experience much the same range of complications but the distribution of their pain is somewhat different. Women have an increased incidence of abdominal and pelvic pain, as well as gynecologic malignancies.

The major difference occurs in psychosocial aspects of the illness. Women with HIV disease tend to be lacking in a well-defined social support network. Many of the patients do not have an extended circle of family or friends who are capable and prepared to be care givers. Many of the women have young children to care for and have little support in raising these children. This presents a significant worry to the patients and a dilemma for health care providers. Fear of losing their children often prevents women from seeking appropriate health care and prevents them from taking opioid medications for adequate pain management.

Once the patients are in an advanced stage of illness requiring institutionalized care, there are few facilities suitable to meet the special needs of these patients. As the number of women with HIV disease has been relatively small until recently, much of the attention and research into meeting the needs of persons with terminal HIV disease is only beginning to address this particular subset of the population.

Research into the problems specific to this population is needed, and resources developed to sensitively care for these patients and provide suitable support to their families and offspring.

CARE OF THE AIDS PATIENT IN THE LAST DAYS OF LIFE

The principles of caring for a patient in the last days include

- the right to die in comfort and dignity.
- continued respect for the patient's wishes.

Management issues to keep in mind:

- Continuous analgesia (buccal, sc, rectal if unable to swallow).
- Continued antiseizure medications if seizures uncontrolled.
- Management of terminal restlessness with benzodiazepine or major tranquilizers (e.g., lorazepam, methotrimeprazine).
- Meticulous attention to comfort measures:
  —mouth care.
  —eye care.
  —nose and lip care.
- Skin care:
  —Frequent turning.
  —Lotion.
- Catheter care.
- Care for family/loved ones:
  —Support.
  —Anticipatory grief.
  —Continued involvement of family/loved ones.
- Continued touching of the patient.
- Continued talking to the patient.

- Someone to be present/nearby, especially if restless.
- Scopolamine for secretions and "death rattle."
- Morphine for dyspnea.
- Religious/ethnic/cultural considerations for the time of death.
- Provisions for family/loved ones to be alone with the body after death.

Suggested Readings

Doyle D, Hanks G, Macdonald N. (eds). Oxford Textbook of Palliative Medicine. Oxford: Oxford University Press, 1993.

Caring Together: The Report of the Expert Working Group on Integrated Palliative Care for Persons With Aids to Health and Welfare Canada Federal Centre for AIDS. Minister of Supply and Services Canada, Ottawa, 1989.

Ferris FD, Flannery JS, McNeal HB, et al. (ed). A Comprehensive Guide for the Care of Persons with HIV Disease, Module 4: Palliative Care. Toronto: Mount Sinai Hospital/Casey House Hospice, 1995.

Foley F (discussion). Pain management in AIDS patients. Pain Manage Newslett 1991;4(3):1–3.

George R. Palliation in AIDS—where do we draw the line? Genitourin Med 1991;67:85–86.

Grothe TM, Brody RV. Palliative care for HIV disease. J Palliat Care 1995;11(2):48–49.

Guidelines on the Termination of Life-Sustaining Treatment and the Care of the Dying: A Report by the Hastings Center. New York: Hastings Center/Indiana University Press, 1987.

Jacox A, Carr DB, Payne R, et al. Management of cancer pain. Clinical practice guideline No. 9. AHCPR Publication No. 94-0592. Rockville, MD: Agency for Health Care Policy and Research, U.S. Department of Health and Human Services, Public Health Service, March 1994.

Kuhl D. Dancing across the lines: People in pain. J Palliat Care 1995;11(2):26–9.

Lobb D. Palliative care for women with AIDS: Identifying the issues. J Palliat Care 1995;11(2):45-7.

Mansfield S, Barter G, Singh S. AIDS and palliative care. Internat J STD AIDS, 1992;3:248–50.

Moss V. Terminal care for people with AIDS. Practitioner, 1991;235:446–9.

Peters B, Beck D, Coleman D, et al. Changing disease pattern in patients with AIDS in a referral centre in the United Kingdom: The changing face of AIDS. Br Med J 1991;302:203–7.

Schofferman J. Care of the terminally ill person with AIDS. Internat Ophthalmol Clin 1989;29(2):127–30.

Schofferman J. Pain: Diagnosis and management in the palliative care of AIDS. J Palliative Care 1988;4(4):46–9.

Sims R, Moss V. Terminal Care for People With AIDS. 2nd ed. London: Edward Arnold, 1994.

Twycross R, Lack S. Therapeutics in Terminal Cancer. 2nd ed. Edinburgh: Churchill Livingstone, 1990.

Ventafridda V, Saita L, Ripamonti C, De Conno F. WHO guidelines for the use of analgesics in cancer pain. Internat J Tissue Reac 1985;7(1):93–6.

von Gunten C, Martinez J, Weitzman S, Von Roenn J. AIDS and hospice. Am J Hospice Palliat Care 1991;July/August:17–9.

Wells RJ. Aspects of palliative care in AIDS. Palliat Med 1987;1:49–52.

The Organization and Integration of Services for Individuals with HIV

R. Scott Rowand

This chapter is designed to outline basic concepts in the planning, organization, and delivery of services for people with HIV infection and AIDS. Geographic and jurisdictional variation in the number of patients, the availability of institutional and community-based resources, and health care financing mechanisms will have a major influence on the design of any system of care.

HIV/AIDS IS A CHRONIC DISEASE

Given an estimated median time from infection to symptom development of 12 years, HIV infection must be considered a relatively indolent chronic disease. Most patients live for several years after an AIDS-defining event, albeit frequently with declining health status. Like other chronic diseases, HIV/AIDS should be considered largely a "primary care disease," with patients supported by specialists only for specific problems or needs.

While patients remain asymptomatic with a relatively intact immune system, care should focus on patient monitoring, health promotion and maintenance, and management of any psychosocial sequelae of a diagnosis of HIV infection. Primary care physicians should be particularly vigilant in the recognition that patients with HIV infections also develop non-HIV-related conditions and health concerns.

With decline in measures of immune system functioning,

264

such as CD4 counts, and/or the appearance of HIV-related complications, clinical intervention and monitoring must increase commensurately. At this stage, it is worthwhile to introduce the patient to the notion of long-term planning related to insurance needs, housing requirements, substitute decision making/living wills, and estate planning. If not already involved, patients may benefit from introduction to an appropriate AIDS service organization (ASO), which can provide practical advice and support. In addition to maximizing health status, services at this stage should be organized in such a way as to encourage independence and continuation of the patient's life-style, including work.

Once patients progress further in their disease and experience more significant decline in health status, the organization and delivery of services becomes an issue of major importance to patients. Seemingly incessant visits to the primary care physicians, specialists, hospitals, numerous laboratories for a variety of diagnostic procedures, pharmacies, welfare agencies, and the like can become physically taxing and demoralizing. At this stage of disease, case management is a valuable approach to improve quality of life for patients.

ORGANIZATION OF A COMPREHENSIVE HIV/AIDS PROGRAM

Under ideal circumstances, care for people living with HIV/AIDS is best organized into a single program by a hospital or health care agency offering a full spectrum of services from primary care through palliative care. A "one-stop shopping" approach, in which the majority of services, including specialist and subspecialist consultation, are provided at one site, reduces the number of locations a patient must visit, improves continuity and coordination of care, allows for maintenance of comprehensive records, and provides an ideal site for the management of clinical trials. Development of care systems in an atmosphere that values research and scholarship not only allows for access to the most current knowledge available but also to therapy in early stages of development. Association of this resource with ASOs, home care providers, and social assistance organizations can further enhance value to patients.

Increasingly, consumers want a voice in decisions that

affect them and the organization and delivery of medical services. Some HIV/AIDS programs have found value in creating community advisory committees, composed of patients, activists, representatives of various ASOs and health care providers, to give guidance and ensure that resources are organized in a manner most acceptable to patients and their community. While governance and management of HIV/AIDS programs must remain vested with the sponsoring organization, there are benefits in creating communication lines and a sense of shared ownership with those affected by HIV/AIDS.

Availability of complementary therapy in association with conventional medical care is controversial. Given the gravity of the disease and the limitations of current therapy, many patients will opt for unconventional approaches. One advantage of a nonjudgmental approach to complementary therapies is the maintenance of an open relationship and the creation of opportunities for observation and monitoring.

CASE MANAGEMENT

Given the multiplicity of resources used by most patients with late-stage disease, case management is a concept that has proven valuable in many settings. Case managers function as service coordinators who facilitate access to needed resources for patients and manage information from multiple sources to assist key providers. A role usually played by nurses or social workers, effective case managers can play a very useful role in eliminating obstacles to care and other frustrations experienced by patients with multiple needs. Data management is especially important to ensure continuity of care.

AIDS SERVICE ORGANIZATIONS

The emergence of AIDS as a significant public health issue in the early 1980s brought with it the establishment of multiple, community-based, ASOs. ASOs act as advocates and frequently offer services based on mutual aid, peer support, and practical assistance. AIDS activists have a record of significant success in influencing public policy and in improving care at the community level. Practitioners involved in care of people with HIV/AIDS should become familiar with ASOs and the services that they offer in order to link patients with such resources, where appropriate.

PROVIDER SUPPORT

Management of patients with HIV/AIDS for many physicians and other health workers is difficult, emotionally draining, less remunerative than other fields of care, and intellectually demanding because of the fast pace of change in information and treatment strategies. Support for physicians and other health care workers, and especially those providing primary care, is crucial.

In many locations, groups of physicians involved in HIV primary care have formed organizations to provide support and continuing education. Use of a "buddy system" that pairs inexperienced physicians with those more knowledgeable about HIV/AIDS has proven helpful. Access to additional clerical resources and physician extenders can assist in filling out the mountain of paper work that accompanies patients enrolled in clinical trials or for health and/or income insurance requirements.

In order to keep abreast of developments in HIV/AIDS, multiple journals and publications are available. Short courses and extended traineeships are offered in many locations. The need to remain current in this rapidly changing field cannot be underestimated, and unless physicians are prepared to make a commitment to the management of this disease and all that goes with it, they are best advised to refer patients to experienced providers.

Other health services providers will also benefit from involvement in association of providers of HIV services. Interest groups have formed for nurses and other professionals at local, regional, and national levels. Offering continuing education, a forum for the presentation of research findings and mutual support, these groups will prove invaluable to the health care professional dedicated to the care of those infected or affected by HIV/AIDS.

Suggested Readings

Cohen PT, Sande MA, Volberg PA. The AIDS Knowledge Base. 2nd ed, chs 4.3, 4.11, 4.15, 4.16, 9.2, 9.3. Boston, Little Brown, 1990.
Cooper S, Weil JA. Developing AIDS inpatient and outpatient services. In Blanchet KD (ed). AIDS: A Health Care Management Response. 1st ed, p. 119. Rockville, MD, Aspen Publishers, 1988.

O'Connor PG, Selwyn PA, Schottenfeld RS. Medical care for injection-drug users with human immunodeficiency virus infection. N Engl J Med 1994; 331: 450–9.

McCormick WC, Inui TS, Deyo RA, et al. Long-term care preferences of hospitalized persons with AIDS. J Gen Intern Med 1991; 6: 524–8.

Wachter RM. AIDS, activism and the politics of health. N Engl J Med 1992; 326: 128–33.

Appendix 1: Adverse Effects of HIV Drugs: Incidence and Management

Alice Tseng, Pharm.D.

Michelle Foisy, Pharm.D.

DRUG	ADVERSE EFFECTS	INCIDENCE (%)	COMMENTS	BASELINE ASSESSMENT, MONITORING
Antiretrovirals Zidovudine (AZT or ZDV; Retrovir)	*CNS:* Headache Malaise	62 53	Transient; may ↓ if start with low dose and titrate up; acetaminophen or NSAID OK	
	GI: Nausea Anorexia Vomiting Hepatomegaly	50 20 17 Rare	Take with nonfatty meal	Baseline LFTs
	Hematologic: Macrocytosis Anemia (<80) Granulocytopenia (<750)	90 1 1.8	R/O folate or B_{12} deficiency Macrocytosis does not respond to B_{12} Dose-related (esp. if >600 mg/d); transfuse if Hgb <75	Can use MCV as measure of compliance Monthly CBC with diff
	Other: Myopathy	10	Related to cumulative dose; D/C drug if Sx, resolution in ~4–8 wks	Often increased CK before symptoms develop
	Nail pigmentation	40	More frequent in blacks	

Drug	Adverse effect	Incidence (%)	Management	Monitoring
Didanosine (ddI; Videx) Dose according to body weight	CNS:			
	Headache	7	Acetaminophen OK to use	
	Fever	12		
	GI:			Amylase, triglycerides
	Pancreatitis	6	Avoid other pancreatoxic agents (see Appendix 3); caution in alcoholics; D/C if ↑ amylase	
	↑ amylase (asymptomatic)	10		
	↑ triglycerides	28		
	Diarrhea	10	Take on empty stomach (consider antiemetic)	
	Abdominal pain			
	Nausea	6		
	MSK:			
	Peripheral neuropathy	20	Related to cumulative use, may improve with ↓ dose or D/C; may also be HIV-related	Baseline neurologic assessment
	Hepatic:			
	↑ AST	13	If LFTs >5x ULN, D/C drug	LFTs
	Liver failure	0.2		
	Lab:			
	Anemia (<80)	2	PRBC transfusion	CBC with diff
	Leukopenia (<2000)	16	D/C if ANC <500 and/or Plts <25,000	
	Thrombocytopenia (<50,000)	2		
	↑ uric acid	2	Do not treat if asymptomatic; D/C if gout	Urate

(Continued)

DRUG	ADVERSE EFFECTS	INCIDENCE (%)	COMMENTS	BASELINE ASSESSMENT, MONITORING
Zalcitabine (ddC; Hivid)	CNS: Headache Myalgia	8 5	Acetaminophen/NSAID	
	GI: Oral ulcers	13	Ulcers reversible with early D/C	R/O non-drug-related causes of oral ulcers
	Dysphagia Abdominal pain	3 3	Take with food if GI upset	
	Pancreatitis	<1	Avoid other pancreatoxic agents (see Appendix 3); caution in alcoholics; D/C if ↑ amylase	Amylase
	Hepatomegaly	<1		LFTs
	MSK: Peripheral neuropathy	17–31	Related to cumulative use, may improve with ↓ dose or D/C May also be HIV-related	Baseline neurologic assessment
	Lab: Anemia (<1500) Leukopenia (<1500) Thrombocytopenia (<50,000) ↑ AST (>250)	5 9 4 5	PRBC transfusion D/C if ANC <500 and/or platelets <25,000 D/C if LFT >5× ULN	CBC with diff LFTs

Drug	Adverse Effects	Incidence (%)	Management
	Other: Rash	8	Consider antihistamine; D/C if no improvement
Stavudine (d4T; Zerit)	*CNS:* Sleep disorders, mania		
	GI: Nausea/vomiting, abdominal pain, diarrhea, pancreatitis	1	Take with food
	Peripheral Neuropathy	15–20	Reversible if D/C
	Other: Neutropenia	3	D/C if ANC <500
	Rash		Consider antihistamine
	↑ LFTs	10	D/C if LFTs >5x ULN
Lamivudine (3TC)	*CNS:* Insomnia, headache		Acetaminophen
	GI: Diarrhea		R/O infectious causes; trial of antidiarrheals; D/C if severe
	Other: Rash, neutropenia		Neutropenia at 20 mg/kg/d; D/C if ANC <500

(Continued)

DRUG	ADVERSE EFFECTS	INCIDENCE (%)	COMMENTS	BASELINE ASSESSMENT, MONITORING
Nevirapine	Rash		Antihistamine	
	Fever		Acetaminophen	
	Thrombocytopenia		D/C if Plt <25,000	
Saquinavir	Headache		Acetaminophen	
	GI disturbances			
Colony-Stimulating Factors				
Granulocyte colony-stimulating factor, G-CSF, filgrastim (Neupogen)	*CNS:*			
	Fever	12	Acetaminophen, diphenhydramine as premedications	
	Fatigue	11		
	Headache	7		
	GI:			
	Nausea, vomiting	57	Dimenhydrinate	
	Diarrhea	14	Antidiarrheal	
	Anorexia	9		
	Other:			
	Bone pain	24	Transient (try acetaminophen/NSAIDs)	
	Alopecia	18		
	Dyspnea	9		
	Skin rash	6	Antihistamine	

	Moderate hypotension	4	Infuse slowly or bolus with 500 cc NS
	Sweet syndrome	1 report	Consider prednisone for Sweet syndrome
	Lab: ↑ uric acid, LDH, ALP	27–58	Do not treat if asymptomatic; D/C if gout	Urate, LFTs
Antivirals Acyclovir (Zovirax)	*Oral Administration:* Diarrhea Vertigo Arthralgia	2.4	Antidiarrheal Meclizine or scopolamine Acetaminophen or NSAID
	IV Administration: Line-Related: Phlebitis	14	Administer more dilute infusion, slow infusion rate, avoid IV infiltration
	CNS: Lethargy, tremors, confusion, seizures	1	Improve in 1–2 weeks; neurotoxicity may clear with hemodialysis; consider anticonvulsants if uncontrolled seizures

(Continued)

DRUG	ADVERSE EFFECTS	INCIDENCE (%)	COMMENTS	BASELINE ASSESSMENT, MONITORING
	Hepatic: ↑ AST, ALT	Rare	D/C if 5x ULN	Baseline LFTs
	Renal: ↑ creatinine hematuria	5	Caution with other nephro-toxins (see Appendix 3) Consider D/C if Scr ↑ >50 mmol/L baseline	Scr, blood urea at baseline then 3x/week Adjust dosage for renal function
Foscarnet (Foscavir)	*CNS:* Mild headache Fatigue Fever Seizures	100 100 25	Consider acetaminophen Often related to ↓ Ca; correct Ca; may consider anticonvulsants for uncontrolled seizures	
	GI: Nausea	80	Consider antiemetic	

Renal/Electrolytes: ↑ creatinine, proteinuria, ↓ K, ↓ Ca, ↓ Mg	33	Caution with other nephrotoxic agents Hydration with 250–500 cc NS pre-postinfusion; infuse slowly via pump to minimize hypocalcemia Slow infusion rate or D/C if periorbal numbing or seizures; obtain ionized serum Ca and correct if needed Supplement lytes as needed	Scr, blood urea, K^+, Ca^{+2}, Mg^{+2}, PO_4^--2–3x/week during induction and q1–2wks during maintenance Adjust dosage for renal function
Lab: ↓ WBC ↓ Hgb ↑ LTFs	<10 <10	D/C if ANC <500 Transfuse if Hgb <75 D/C if LFTs >5x ULN	CBC, diff 2–3x/week during induction and q1–2wks during maintenance LFTs
Other: Neuropathy Penile ulcers		Caution with other neurotoxic agents (e.g., ddI, ddC, INH) Hydrate well, urinate frequently, good hygiene; usually reversible if D/C drug	

(Continued)

DRUG	ADVERSE EFFECTS	INCIDENCE (%)	COMMENTS	BASELINE ASSESSMENT, MONITORING
Ganciclovir (Cytovene)	*Hematologic:* Granulocytopenia Thrombocytopenia Anemia	40 20 2	Caution with other hematosuppressants Dose-related; may respond to G-CSF	CBC with diff q2d during induction, and at least once weekly thereafter
	Other: Fever, rash	2	Acetaminophen Diphenhydramine	
Antifungals Amphotericin B (Fungizone)	*Infusion-Related:* Phlebitis, rigors, fever	Common	Premedication (acetaminophen 650 mg, hydrocortisone 25mg, meperidine, ibuprofen) Infuse over 4–6 hours; tolerance develops over time; D/C if cardiac Sx	Baseline Na, K, renal, cardiac function; Monitor vital signs during infusion
	Hypotension, ventricular fibrillation	Less frequent		
	GI: Nausea, vomiting, anorexia, metallic taste, abdominal pain		Antiemetic Sometimes subside with continued administration	

Drug / Adverse Effect	Incidence	Management	Monitoring
Renal: ↑ creatinine, nephrocalcinosis, renal tubular acidosis	80 Rare	Not renally eliminated, but may need to ↓ dose or hold to minimize renal toxicity if Scr >230 µmol/L	Hydration, Na loading Scr, blood urea 2–3x/weekly
Lab: ↓ K, ↓ Mg, anemia	Common	K, Mg suppl. Transfuse if Hgb <75	Mg, K, urinalysis, CBC 2–3x/week
Fluconazole (Diflucan)			
CNS: Headache	1.9	Acetaminophen	
GI: Nausea	3.7	Take with food	
Abdominal pain	1.7		
Vomiting	1.7	Antiemetic	
Diarrhea	1.5	Antidiarrheal	
Hepatic: ↑ AST	20	D/C drug if LFTs >5x ULN	LFTs
Severe hepatotoxicity	Rare		
Skin: Rash	1.8	Antihistamine	
Exfoliative dermatitis	Rare	D/C if exfoliative	

(Continued)

DRUG	ADVERSE EFFECTS	INCIDENCE (%)	COMMENTS	BASELINE ASSESSMENT, MONITORING
Flucytosine (Ancotil)	*GI:* Diarrhea, anorexia, nausea, vomiting	6	Antiemetic	
	Hematologic: Leukopenia, thrombocytopenia Aplastic anemia	22 Rare	Especially when serum level >100 µg/mL; adjust dose in renal failure (caution with concurrent nephrotoxins)	Measure serum levels
Ketoconazole (Nizoral)	*GI:* Nausea, vomiting	3	Can take with food; consider antiemetics	
	Hepatic: ↑ AST Hepatotoxicity	2–5 Rare	D/C if >5x ULN	LFTs
	Other: Fever, rash, gynecomastia, ↓ testosterone and corticosteroid synthesis, reversible adrenal insufficiency, impotence, ↓ libido	3–8	Acetaminophen, diphenhydramine D/C if symptoms severe	Symptoms of adrenal suppression

Itraconazole (Sporanox)			
CNS:			
Headache	4	Acetaminophen	
CV:			
Hypertension	3	Low-Na diet; D/C if severe	BP
GI:			
Nausea	11	Can take with food, consider antiemetic	
Vomiting	5		
Diarrhea	3	Antidiarrheal	
Hepatic:			
↑ LFTs	3	D/C if >5x ULN	LFTs
Hepatitis	Rare		
Skin:			
Rash	9	Consider antihistamine	
Pruritis	3		
Other:			
Edema	4	Low-Na diet?	Evidence of edema
Fever	3	Acetaminophen	
Lab:			
↓ K	7	Replace K; caution with other K-wasting agents (see Appendix 3)	Electrolytes

(Continued)

DRUG	ADVERSE EFFECTS	INCIDENCE (%)	COMMENTS	BASELINE ASSESSMENT, MONITORING
Antimycobacterials Amikacin (Amikin) 15 mg/kg/d IV (use corrected BW if obese)	CNS: Ototoxicity (high frequency)		Monitor serum concentrations Desired peak 35–45, trough <4 D/C if problematic Caution with other ototoxins	Bimonthly serial audiograms if prolonged therapy Monitor for vertigo, dizziness, hearing loss, nausea Monitor drug levels
	MSK: Neuromuscular blockade	Animal studies	Caution with neuromuscular blockers, myasthenia, botulism, parkinsonism; infuse over 1 hour	
	Renal: Nephrotoxicity		Dose adjustment in renal failure; caution with other nephrotoxins	Scr, blood urea Monitor drug levels
Azithromycin (Zithromax)	CNS: Ototoxicity	≤17	↑ with high doses (≥600 mg/d) for prolonged duration; slowly reversible upon D/C	

Drug	Adverse Effects	Incidence	Management	Monitoring
	GI: Diarrhea	4	Should be taken on empty stomach for best absorption	
	Nausea	3	Consider antiemetic/antidiarrheal	
	Abdominal pain	2		
	Vomiting	1		
	Lab: ↑ AST	1.5	D/C if LFTs >5x ULN	LFTs
	Hepatotoxicity	Rare		
Capreomycin sulfate (Capastat)	*CNS:* Ototoxicity	11		Audiometry
	MSK: Neuromuscular Blockade	Partial with large doses	Enhanced by ether analgesia Antagonized by neostigmine	
	Renal: Nephrotoxicity	36		Scr, BUN
Ciprofloxacin (Cipro)	*CNS:* Headache, insomnia	0.4	Acetaminophen	
	GI: Nausea, diarrhea, vomiting, abdominal pain	1.5	Take with food (avoid antacids)	
	Skin: Rash	0.6	Antihistamine	

(Continued)

DRUG	ADVERSE EFFECTS	INCIDENCE (%)	COMMENTS	BASELINE ASSESSMENT, MONITORING
	Lab:			
	↑ AST	1.7	D/C if LFTs >5× ULN	LFTs
	↑ ALP	0.8		
	↓ WBC	0.4	D/C if ANC <500	CBC with diff
	Other:			
	Cartilage erosion in animals	?	If possible, avoid in children/ pregnant women	
Clarithromycin (Biaxin)	*CNS:*			
	Headache	2	Acetaminophen	
	Ototoxicity	Rare	D/C if hearing loss occurs	
	GI:			
	Diarrhea	3	Take with food	
	Nausea	3		
	Abnormal taste	3		
	Abdominal pain	2		
	Dyspepsia	2		
	Lab:			
	↑ AST, ALP	<1	D/C if >5× ULN	LFTs
	Eye:			
	Conjunctival irritation, retinal crystal deposition	<1	D/C if Sx	

Drug	Adverse effects	Incidence (%)	Management
Clofazimine (Lamprene)	*GI:* Abdominal pain	50	Take with food
	Skin: Pink-brown-black pigmentation	75–100	Topical emollient
	Dryness	20	Antihistamine
	Pruritus	5	
Cycloserine (Seromycin)	*CNS:* Convulsions, psychoses	5–10	↑ with ↑ dose; give 50 mg pyridoxine for every 250 mg cycloserine daily
Ethambutol (Myambutol)	*CNS:* Optic neuritis with ↓ visual acuity, central scotomata, loss of green and red perception	<6	Neuritis ↑ with doses >15 mg/kg/d Do not exceed dosage of 25 mg/kg/d Usually reversible if D/C drug Periodic evaluation of visual acuity (>10% loss = significant) if on long-term therapy
	Other: Rash, arthralgia, hyperuricemia, anaphylactoid reaction	Rare	Antihistamine Acetaminophen

(Continued)

DRUG	ADVERSE EFFECTS	INCIDENCE (%)	COMMENTS	BASELINE ASSESSMENT, MONITORING
Ethionamide (Trecator-SC)	*GI:* GI irritation, stomatitis	<50%	Dose-related; give with meals/antacids	
	Hepatic: Hepatitis	Rare		LFTs
	Peripheral neuropathy	Rare	50–100 mg pyridoxine daily	
Isoniazid	Peripheral neuropathy	<1	Rx pyridoxine 25–50 mg daily	
	Allergic: Rashes, fever	Rare	Usually within 6–7 weeks Antihistamine or D/C and restart at lower dose	
	Other: Hepatitis	10–15	Acetaminophen D/C if LFTs >5x ULN	LFTs
Para-aminosalicylic acid (PAS) (Tebrazide)	*GI:* GI irritation	10–15	Take with food	
	Other: Hepatitis, arthralgia, myalgia, rashes, drug fever		D/C if LFTs >5x ULN Acetaminophen Antihistamine	LFTs

Pyrazinamide	*GI:* Gastric irritation		Take with food	
	Hepatic: Hepatitis	2	Do not exceed 25 mg/kg/d	LFTs
	Other: Arthralgia, hyperuricemia		Acetaminophen	Urate
Rifabutin (Mycobutin)	*CNS:* Uveitis	1	Dose-related; reversible with D/C of drug, may restart lower dose	
	Insomnia	1		
	GI: Nausea	6	Take with food	
	Abdominal pain	4		
	Diarrhea	3		
	Hematologic: Leukopenia	17	D/C if ANC <500	CBC with diff monthly
	Thrombocytopenia	5	D/C if Plt <25,000	
	Skin: Rash, orange-tan pigmentation	11	Antihistamine	
	Lab: ↑ AST/ALT	8	D/C if >5x ULN	LFTs
	Other: Fever	2	Acetaminophen	
	Discolored (reddish) urine	30		

(Continued)

DRUG	ADVERSE EFFECTS	INCIDENCE (%)	COMMENTS	BASELINE ASSESSMENT, MONITORING
Rifampin (Rifadin)	*GI:*			
	GI irritation		Take with food	
	Hematologic:			
	Thrombocytopenia	1	D/C if Plt <25,000	CBC with diff
	Leukopenia	1	D/C if ANC <500	
	Hemolytic anemia	Rare		
	Hepatic:			
	↑ LFTs			LFTs
	Jaundice	Rare	D/C if LFTs >5x ULN	
	Other:			
	Drug fever	1		
	Anaphylactoid reactions			
	Flu syndrome			
	Pruritis ± rash	1	Antihistamine	
	Orange-brown discoloration of body fluids		Caution with contact lenses	
Streptomycin	*CNS:*			
	Vestibular dysfunction (vertigo), dizziness, nausea, tinnitus			
	High frequency loss	1		

Antiparasitic Drugs
Atovaquone (Mepron)

Adverse effect	Incidence	Management
Renal:		
Nephrotoxicity	Rare	Scr, blood urea
Other:		
Allergic skin rashes	4–5	Antihistamine
Drug fever		Acetaminophen
CNS:		
Headache	16	Acetaminophen
Insomnia	10	
Dizziness	3	
General:		
Fever	14	
GI:		
Nausea	21	Take with fatty meal
Diarrhea	19	Consider antidiarrheal
Vomiting	14	
Abdominal pain	4	
Skin:		
Rash	23	Antihistamine
Pruritus	5	

(Continued)

DRUG	ADVERSE EFFECTS	INCIDENCE (%)	COMMENTS	BASELINE ASSESSMENT, MONITORING
	Lab:			
	Anemia (Hgb <80)	6	Transfuse if Hgb <75	CBC with diff
	Neutropenia (<750)	3	D/C if ANC <500	
	↑ AST	4	D/C if LFTs >5× ULN	LFTs
	↑ Amylase	7		
Clindamycin (Dalacin)	*GI:*			
	Diarrhea, nausea	<3	Culture for *C. difficile* toxin	
	Skin:			
	Rash		Antihistamine	
	Lab:			
	Neutropenia		D/C if ANC <500	CBC with diff
Dapsone (Avlosulfon)	*GI:*			CBC
	Nausea, vomiting, oral lesions			
	Hematologic:			
	Hemolytic anemia		↑ if G6PD deficient	
	Methemoglobinemia		Check for methemoglobinemia if pt dyspneic; D/C if >10–15%	
	Skin:			
	Allergic rash (30%) cross-reactivity with sulfas)		Can try to "treat through" with antihistamine, or may consider desensitization	

Metronidazole (Flagyl)	*CNS:* Headache, paresthesias, disulfiram-like reaction		Avoid alcohol during/48 hours post-treatment	
	GI: Nausea, vomiting, metallic taste		Take with food	
	Other: Dark urine, tears, sweat		Harmless	
Paramomycin (Humatin)	*CNS:* Vertigo, headache		Meclizine, scopolamine Acetaminophen	
	GI: Nausea, abdominal cramps, diarrhea, pancreatitis	Rare	Usually with doses >3 g	Amylase
	Skin: Rash		Antihistamine	
Pentamidine isethionate IV	*Infusion-Related:* Hypotension, arrhythmias	9.6	Infuse slowly over min. 1 hour Prehydrate with 500 cc NS bolus	Monitor vital signs during infusion

(Continued)

DRUG	ADVERSE EFFECTS	INCIDENCE (%)	COMMENTS	BASELINE ASSESSMENT, MONITORING
	GI:			
	Nausea, vomiting	8.2	Antiemetic	
	Pancreatitis	<1	Avoid other pancreatoxins	Amylase
	Renal:			
	Nephrotoxicity	23	Caution with other nephrotoxins	Scr, blood urea
	Skin:			
	Rash	1.5	Antihistamine	
	Lab:			
	Neutropenia	15	D/C if ANC <500 or Plt <25,000	CBC with diff
	Thrombocytopenia	4		
	Hypoglycemia, followed by hyperglycemia	6.2	If blood glucose <3 mmol/L consider D50W Hyperglycemia may result in IDDM	Blood glucose
	↓ Ca, ↑ K, ↓ Mg		Supplement as required; Kayexalate for hyperkalemia	Electrolytes
Pentamidine aerosol	*Resp:*			
	Cough, bronchospasm	15–38	Bronchodilator	
	Pneumothorax	1–5		

(Continued)

Primaquine	*Hematologic:* Hemolytic anemia Methemoglobinemia	Rare	Esp. if G6PD-deficient	CBC with diff
Pyrimethamine (Daraprim)	*GI:* Vomiting, diarrhea Xerostomia *Hematologic:* Megaloblastic anemia, neutropenia, thrombocytopenia *Skin:* Rash	Common Rare 25	Take with food Give folinic acid 10–50 mg/d Antihistamine	CBC with diff
Sulfadiazine	*Allergic:* Rash, fever, pruritus, photo- sensitization, Stevens-John- son syndrome *GI:* Nausea, vomiting *Hematologic:* Blood dyscrasias (usually agranulocytosis) Hemolytic anemia		Try antihistamine, consider desensitization regimen, or D/C Antiemetic D/C if ANC <500 In G6PD deficient	CBC with diff

DRUG	ADVERSE EFFECTS	INCIDENCE (%)	COMMENTS	BASELINE ASSESSMENT, MONITORING
Trimethoprim (Proloprim)	*Hepatic:* Hepatic toxicity *Renal:* Crystalluria		D/C if LFTs >5× ULN Drink with full glass of water	LFTs
	Hematologic: Marrow suppression *Skin:* Rash, pruritus	Rare <TMP-SMX		CBC with diff
Trimethoprim-sulfameth-oxazole (TMP-SMX) (Bactrim, Septra)	*Allergic:* Rash, fever	High	Typically occurs at day 10–14, but may occur at any time (days–months) Rash often preceded by fever Often dose-related; can try to "treat through" with antihistamines, or may consider desensitization	

Hematologic:			
Bone marrow suppression		D/C if ANC <500	CBC with diff
Hepatic:			
↑ LFTs		D/C if LFTs >5× ULN	LFTs
Hepatotoxicity	Rare		
Lab:			
↑ K		Due to high-dose TMP (i.e., 15–20 mg/kg/d); consider Kayexalate	Electrolytes
Trimetrexate (Neutrexin)			
Allergic:			
Rash	3	Antihistamine	
Fever	2	Antipyretic	
Hematologic:			
Neutropenia (<1000)	4	Must administer with folinic acid	CBC with diff
Thrombocytopenia		D/C if ANC <500 or Plt <25,000	
Hepatic:			
↑ AST	3	D/C if LFTs >5× ULN	LFTs

(Continued)

DRUG	ADVERSE EFFECTS	INCIDENCE (%)	COMMENTS	BASELINE ASSESSMENT, MONITORING
Appetite Stimulants				
Dronabinol (Marinol)	*CNS:* Elation, laughing, dizziness, confusion, paranoid reactions Somnolence	8 3–10	Dose-related	
	GI: Nausea, vomiting		Antiemetic	
Megestrol acetate (Megace)	*CNS:* Excitation *GI:* Diarrhea, flatulence *Other:* Impotence, rash, edema, hyperglycemia		Antidiarrheal ↓ dose or D/C Antihistamine for rash	Blood glucose

Appendix 2: Drug Desensitization Protocols

Alice Tseng, Pharm.D.

Michelle Foisy, Pharm.D.

TRIMETHOPRIM-SULFAMETHOXAZOLE (SEPTRA) DESENSITIZATION

1-Day Oral Protocol*

1. Admit to clinic:

- NPO during initial period.
- Take vital signs on admission and discharge.
- Pharmacy to provide trimethoprim-sulfamethoxazole (TMP-SMX) doses, determined by the SMX component (compounding instructions follow).

2. Give TMP-SMX as follows:

- q15 min: 1 µg, 10 µg, 50 µg, 100 µg, 500 µg, 1.0 mg
- then q30 min: 2 mg, 5 mg, 10 mg, 50 mg, 100 mg
- 4 hours later: Septra tablet (400 mg)

3. Discharge home if stable.

4. Commencing next day: Septra DS (800 mg) daily. On occasion, the patient takes regular-strength Septra for 1 week then Septra DS.

5. All available for IV use: epinephrine, methylprednisolone sodium succinate (Solu-Medrol), diphenhydramine (Benadryl), ranitidine (Zantac).

---

*Developed by Richard Fralick, M.D., F.R.C.P.C., C.C.F.P., M.H.Sc., The Wellesley Hospital, Toronto, ON.

Compounding Instructions

STEP 1. Take 40 ml of Septra suspension (200 mg SMX/40 mg TMP per 5 ml) and qs to 80 ml with distilled water to make **20 mg SMX/ml suspension** (1:1 dilution). Shake well.

STEP 2. Take 10 ml of the 1:1 dilution (from Step 1) and qs to 100 ml with distilled water to make a **2 mg SMX/ml suspension** (1:10 dilution). Shake well.

For protocol, dispense as follows:

2 mg SMX (1 ml), 5 mg SMX (2.5 ml), 10 mg SMX (5 ml), 50 mg SMX (25 ml), 100 mg SMX (50 ml).

STEP 3. Take 10 ml of the 1:10 dilution (from Step 2) and qs to 100 ml with distilled water to make a **0.2 mg SMX/ml suspension** (1:100 dilution). Shake well.

STEP 4. Take 10 ml of the 1:100 dilution (from Step 3) and qs to 100 ml with distilled water to make a **0.02 mg SMX/ml suspension** (1:1000 dilution). Shake well.

For protocol, dispense as follows:

50 µg (2.5 ml), 100 µg (5 ml), 500 µg (25 ml), 1 mg (50 ml).

STEP 5. Take 10 ml of the 1:1000 dilution (from Step 4) and qs to 100 ml with distilled water to make a **0.002 mg SMX/ml suspension** (1:10,000 dilution). Shake well.

For protocol, dispense as follows:

1 µg (0.5 ml), 10 µg (5 ml)

Shake well before using; keep suspensions refrigerated.

2-Day Oral Protocol*

1. Admit to clinic:

- NPO during initial period.
- Take vital signs on admission and discharge.
- Pharmacy to provide trimethoprim-sulfamethoxazole (TMP-SMX) doses, determined by the SMX component (compounding instructions are as for 1-day protocol, but make double the amount of 1:10 dilution).
- *Day 1:* Give TMP-SMX as follows:
- q15 min: 1 µg, 10 µg, 100 µg, 500 µg, 1.0 mg
- then q30 min: 2 mg, 5 mg, 10 mg, 50 mg
- *Day 2:* Give TMP-SMX as follows:

---

*Developed by Richard Fralick, M.D., F.R.C.P.C., C.C.F.P., M.H.Sc., The Wellesley Hospital, Toronto, ON.

- q30 min: 50 mg, 75 mg, 100 mg
- 4 hours later: Septra tablet (400 mg)

2. Discharge home if stable.

3. Commencing next day: Septra DS (800 mg) daily. On occasion, the patient takes regular-strength Septra for 1 week then Septra DS.

All available for IV use: epinephrine, methylprednisolone sodium succinate (Solu-Medrol), diphenhydramine (Benadryl), ranitidine (Zantac).

8-Day Oral Protocol*

One double-strength tablet, trimethoprim 160 mg and sulfamethoxazole 800 mg, is the drug of choice in primary and secondary *Pneumocystis carinii* pneumonia prophylaxis. The incidence of cutaneous reactions to TMP-SMX in hospitalized patients has been reported to be as high as 3.3. percent, however, in HIV-positive patients, the range is 40 to 80 percent. The symptoms of these hypersensitivity reactions have included fever, morbilliform eruption, pruritus, headache, malaise, and myalgia. Other adverse effects have included elevated liver function tests and neutropenia. In some instances, patients have experienced life-threatening reactions, including anaphylaxis and Stevens–Johnson syndrome. We have developed a protocol and successfully desensitized 56 out of 61 HIV-positive patients (92 percent) to TMP-SMX, using an oral method.

The procedure is completed over 8 days with doses of TMP-SMX q6h. Solutions are made from standard oral suspension (40 mg TMP/200 mg SMX per 5 ml). The final concentrations of TMP and SMX and the dilutions are as follows:

Day 1: 0.000004 mg TMP/0.00002 mg SMX per 1 ml (1:1,000,000 dilution)

1 ml

2 ml

4 ml

8 ml

Day 2: 0.00004 mg TMP/0.0002 mg SMX per 1 ml (1:100,000 dilution)

1 ml

2 ml

---

*Developed by Conant MA, and Allen B. Oral desensitization to trimethoprim-sulfamethoxazole (8-day regimen), reprinted by permission.

4 ml

8 ml

Day 3: 0.0004 mg TMP/0.002 mg SMX per 1 ml (1:10,000 dilution)

1 ml

2 ml

4 ml

8 ml

Day 4: 0.004 mg TMP/0.02 mg SMX per 1 ml (1:1000 dilution)

1 ml

2 ml

4 ml

8 ml

Day 5: 0.04 mg TMP/0.2 mg SMX per 1 ml (1:100 dilution)

1 ml

2 ml

4 ml

8 ml

Day 6: 0.4 mg TMP/2.0 mg SMX per 1 ml (1:10 dilution)

1 ml

2 ml

4 ml

8 ml

Day 7: 4.0 mg TMP/20.0 mg SMX per 1 ml (1:1 dilution)

1 ml

2 ml

4 ml

8 ml

Day 8: 8.0 mg TMP/40.0 mg SMX per 1 ml (standard oral suspension)

5 ml

10 ml

20 ml

Last dose: 1 DS tablet

Following Day 8: 1 DS tablet qd.

At the onset of a drug reaction at any time during desensitization, patients should call their primary care provider. For the following symptoms we recommend the corresponding treatments:

Low-grade fever, malaise, myalgia	Aspirin or Tylenol q4h prn
Mild morbilliform eruption	Diphenhydramine hydro-chloride (Benadryl) 25–50 mg q6–8 h prn; 50 mg hs

Raging fever and/or florid morbilliform eruption	Prednisone
	20 mg TID for 3 days
	15 mg TID for 3 days
	10 mg TID for 3 days
	10 mg once a day for 3 days

Management Suggestions

- The first dose of TMP-SMX should be administered in the office, and patients should be observed for anaphylaxis for 1 hour.

- Each patient should have a home monitor, someone who can observe the patient after each dose and summon help if anaphylaxis occurs.

- Instruct patients to drink 3000 ml of fluids daily.

- Instruct patients to use a sunscreen with SPF 15.

- Instruct patients not to interrupt therapy, even for 1 or 2 days, because allergic reaction may occur.

- Finally, frequent calls to patients and necessary office visits to provide supervision and encouragement appear beneficial to a successful outcome.

Compounding Instructions

STEP 1. Start with commercially available Septra suspension containing 40 mg TMP and 200 mg SMX per 5 ml. Dispense 60 ml and label as bottle for Day 8.

STEP 2. Take 40 ml Septra suspension and qs to 80 ml with distilled water. The resulting suspension contains 20 mg SMX per ml (1:1 dilution). Shake well. Dispense 60 ml and label as bottle for Day 7.

STEP 3. Take 10 ml of 1:1 dilution (from step 2) and qs to 100 ml with distilled water. The resulting suspension contains 2 mg SMX per ml (1:10 dilution). Shake well. Dispense 60 ml and label as bottle for Day 6.

STEP 4. Take 10 ml of 1:10 dilution (from step 3) and qs to 100 ml with distilled water. The resulting suspension contains 0.2 mg SMX per ml (1:100 dilution). Shake well. Dispense 60 ml and label as bottle for Day 5.

STEP 5. Take 10 ml of 1:100 dilution (from step 4) and qs to 100 ml with distilled water. The resulting suspension contains 0.02 mg SMX per ml (1:1,000 dilution). Shake well. Dispense 60 ml and label as bottle for Day 4.

STEP 6. Take 10 ml of 1:1,000 dilution (from step 5) and qs to 100 ml with distilled water. The resulting suspension contains 0.002 mg SMX per ml (1:10,000 dilution). Shake well. Dispense 60 ml and label as bottle for Day 3.

STEP 7.   Take 10 ml of 1:10,000 dilution (from step 6) and qs to 100 ml with distilled water. The resulting suspension contains 0.0002 mg SMX per ml (1:100,000 dilution). Shake well. Dispense 60 ml and label as bottle for Day 2.

STEP 8.   Take 10 ml of 1:100,000 dilution (from step 7) and qs to 100 ml with distilled water. The resulting suspension contains 0.00002 mg SMX per ml (1:1,000,000 dilution). Shake well. Dispense 60 ml and label as bottle for Day 1.

Dispensing Instructions

STEP 1.   Dispense one 60 ml (2 oz.) bottle of each diluted suspension and an oral syringe for each of the 8 days of the protocol.

STEP 2.   Label each bottle of diluted suspension with appropriate concentration and quantity of SMX mL. For example:

Bottle #2. 1:100,000 dilution.

Each cc contains: 0.00004 mg TMP and 0.0002 mg SMX.

STEP 3.   Label each bottle with the day and dosage regimen as follows:

DAYS #1-7	DAY #8
Take 1 ml at 6:00 am	Take 5 ml at 6:00 am
Take 2 ml at 12:00 noon	Take 10 ml at 12:00 noon
Take 4 ml at 6:00 pm	Take 20 ml at 6:00 pm
Take 8 ml at 12:00 midnight	Take one DS tablet at 12:00 midnight

Note: These instructions should go on each bottle. The instructions are the same for Days 1–7, only the concentration of the suspension changes. Day 8 different doses are used.

STEP 4.   Label each bottle *"Shake Well Before Using"* and *"Keep Refrigerated."* Stability 4 to 6 weeks. No concern about stability if prepared properly.

Patient Instructions:

STEP 1.   Shake the bottle thoroughly before each dose.

STEP 2.   Following the midnight dose discard the bottle and syringe used during that day.

STEP 3.   Drink 3 L (approx. eight 12-ounce glasses) of fluid daily while on the protocol.

STEP 4.   Use sunscreen with SPF 15 before going out into the sun.

IV Protocol*

1. Solutions needed:

- Septra 10 mg in D_5W 100 ml (i.e., 2 minims in 1000 ml)
- Septra 1 g in D_5W 1000 ml (i.e., 12.5 cc's in 1000 ml)

2. Admit to clinic:

- Take vital signs on admission.
- Start IV with D_5W TKVO.

3. Give Septra solution #1 q15 min IV push as follows:

- 1 ml over 1 minute
- 2 ml over 1.5 minutes
- 5 ml over 3 minutes
- 10 ml over 5 minutes
- 20 ml over 8 minutes
- 50 ml over 10 minutes

4. Give Septra solution #2 q30 min as follows:

- 1 ml over 1 minute, IV push
- 5 ml over 2 minutes, IV push
- 20 ml over 5 minutes via AVI pump
- 50 ml over 10 minutes via AVI pump
- 100 ml over 15 minutes via AVI pump
- 250 ml over 20 minutes via AVI pump

5. One hour later give Septra (400 mg) tablet PO.
6. Flush line with D_5W; if no adverse effect, disconnect IV and discharge patient.
7. Commencing next day: Septra DS (800 mg) daily.

DAPSONE DESENSITIZATION
1-Day Oral Protocol*

1. Administer dapsone doses as follows:

- q 15 min: 1 µg, 5 µg, 10 µg, 50 µg, 100 µg, 200 µg, 500 µg, 1 mg PO
- q 30 min: 2 mg, 5 mg, 10 mg, 50 mg PO

Developed by Richard Fralick, M.D., F.R.C.P.C., C.C.F.P., M.H.Sc., The Wellesley Hospital, Toronto, ON.

2. Then, dapsone 100 mg PO daily from next day.

3. Measure vital signs on admission and q2h if stable.

Compounding Instructions

STEP 1.   Crush 100-mg dapsone tablet, qs to 1000 mg with lactose to make 100 mg dapsone/1000 mg mixture.

- Make 1: 10 mg dapsone/100 mg capsule
- Make 1: 5 mg dapsone/50 mg capsule

STEP 2.   Take 100 mg of mixture from Step 1 (i.e., 10 mg dapsone), qs to 1000 mg with lactose.

- Make 3: 1 mg dapsone/100 mg capsule
- Make 1: 0.5 mg dapsone/50 mg capsule

STEP 3.   Take 100 mg of mixture from Step 2 (i.e., 1 mg dapsone), qs to 1000 mg with lactose.

- Make 3: 0.1 mg dapsone/100 mg capsule
- Make 1: 50 µg dapsone/50 mg capsule

STEP 4.   Take 100 mg of mixture from Step 3 (i.e., 0.1 mg dapsone), qs to 1000 mg with lactose.

- Make 1: 10 µg dapsone/100 mg capsule
- Make 1: 5 µg dapsone/50 mg capsule

STEP 5.   Take 100 mg of mixture from Step 4 (i.e., 10 µg dapsone), qs to 1000 with lactose.

- Make 1: 1 µg dapsone/100 mg capsule

14-Day Oral Protocol*

NB: this protocol has not yet been administered in clinical practice.

Day Number	Daily Oral Dose
1	0.01 mg OD (solution from tablets)
2	0.01 mg BID
3	0.1 mg OD
4	0.1 mg BID
5	1.0 mg OD
6	1.0 mg BID
7	2.0 mg BID

Adapted from Metroka CE et al., JAMA 1992;267:512, copyright 1992, American Medical Assoc., by Brian M. Cornelson, M.D., C.C.F.P., The Wellesley Hospital, Toronto, ON., reprinted by permission.

8	4.0 mg BID
9	8.0 mg BID
10	16.0 mg BID
11	25.0 mg BID
12	35.0 mg BID
13	45.0 mg BID
14	50.0 mg BID (whole tablets)

PENTAMIDINE DESENSITIZATION

Aerosol Protocol*

Dilution	Volume Inhaled (ml)	Amount Delivered (mg)
1:10,000	4	0.006
1:1000	4	0.06
1:100	4	0.6
1:10	4	6
Full strength	20	300

IV Protocol†

Dilution	Volume Infused (ml) (in 15-minute intervals)	Amount Delivered (mg)
1:10,000	2	0.00016
1:1000	2	0.0016
1:100	2	0.016
1:10	2	0.16
Full strength	250 (in 2 hours)	200

*Adapted from Baum et al. J Allergy Clin Immunol 1992;90(2): 268–9.

†Adapted from Greenberger et al. J Allergy Clin Immunol 1987;79:484–8.

SULFADIAZINE DESENSITIZATION

6 Day Oral Protocol*

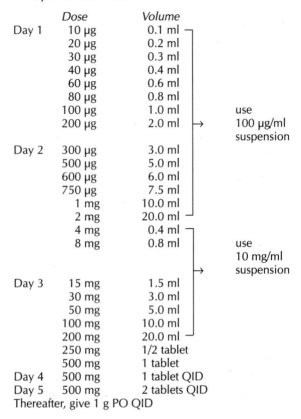

	Dose	*Volume*	
Day 1	10 µg	0.1 ml	
	20 µg	0.2 ml	
	30 µg	0.3 ml	
	40 µg	0.4 ml	
	60 µg	0.6 ml	
	80 µg	0.8 ml	
	100 µg	1.0 ml	use
	200 µg	2.0 ml	→ 100 µg/ml suspension
Day 2	300 µg	3.0 ml	
	500 µg	5.0 ml	
	600 µg	6.0 ml	
	750 µg	7.5 ml	
	1 mg	10.0 ml	
	2 mg	20.0 ml	
	4 mg	0.4 ml	
	8 mg	0.8 ml	use 10 mg/ml suspension
Day 3	15 mg	1.5 ml	→
	30 mg	3.0 ml	
	50 mg	5.0 ml	
	100 mg	10.0 ml	
	200 mg	20.0 ml	
	250 mg	1/2 tablet	
	500 mg	1 tablet	
Day 4	500 mg	1 tablet QID	
Day 5	500 mg	2 tablets QID	

Thereafter, give 1 g PO QID

- for Days 1–3, administer oral doses q3h.
- concurrent medications:
    - —pyrimethamine 25 mg BID
    - —folinic acid 7.5 mg daily
    - —clindamycin 300 mg QID (discontinue once desensitization complete)

As described by Tenant-Flowers et al. AIDS 1991;5:311–5, Rapid Science Publishers; reprinted by permission.

DAY	BOTTLE	DILUTION	CONCENTRATION (TMP COMPONENT IN MG/ML)	CONCENTRATION (SMX COMPONENT IN MG/ML)
1	1	1:1,000,000	0.000004	0.00002
2	2	1:100,000	0.00004	0.0002
3	3	1:10,000	0.0004	0.002
4	4	1:1,000	0.004	0.02
5	5	1:100	0.04	0.2
6	6	1:10	0.4	2.0
7	7	1:1	4.0	20
8	8	standard suspension	8.0	40

Appendix 3: Drug–Drug Interactions

Michelle Foisy, Pharm.D.

Alice Tseng, Pharm.D.

DRUGS	CONCOMITANT DRUG	COMMON SIDE EFFECTS/TOXICITY	COMMENTS	MONITORING
Antiretrovirals ddC (dideoxycytidine, zalcitabine, HIVID)	*Neurotoxins:* Dapsone, ethionamide, isoniazid, metronidazole, nitrofurantoin, phenytoin, cisplatin, vincristine	↑ risk of neuropathy	Caution with combination of listed medications.	
	Pancreatoxins: ddI, ethanol, pentamidine, valproic acid	↑ risk of pancreatitis	Avoid combination of ddI and ddC. Discontinue ddC therapy throughout and for 1 week after pentamidine IV for acute PCP treatment. Avoid ddC in those with a history of ethanol abuse and/or pancreatitis.	Amylase, lipase monthly.
	Trimethoprim	↑ AUC of ddC 37%	May increase risk of ddC-associated toxicities.	Monitor for ddC toxicities.

(Continued)

DRUGS	CONCOMITANT DRUG	COMMON SIDE EFFECTS/TOXICITY	COMMENTS	MONITORING
ddI (dideoxyinosine, didanosine, Videx)			To ↑ absorption, formulation contains Al³⁺/Mg²⁺ buffer, which may cause interactions via alteration of pH or cation chelation. ddI should be taken on an empty stomach.	
	Ketoconazole, itraconazole capsules, quinolones (ciprofloxacin, ofloxacin), tetracycline	ddI causes ↓ absorption of agents listed	Agents listed should be taken at least 2 hours before or after ddI. It is preferable to give ddI 6 hours before or 2 hours after quinolones.	Monitor for efficacy of listed agents.
	Ganciclovir	*With PO ganciclovir:* ↑ ddI conc. >100%; ↓ GCV conc. 20% with sequential administration *With IV ganciclovir:* ↑ ddI conc. >70%	Potential for ↑ ddI toxicity and ↓ ganciclovir efficacy. Administer oral ganciclovir before/with ddI to minimize effect on ganciclovir absorption.	Monitor for ddI toxicity and progression of CMV disease.
	Neurotoxins	↑ risk neurotoxicity	See ddC	See ddC
	Pancreatoxins	↑ risk pancreatitis	See ddC	See ddC

Zidovudine (AZT, Retrovir)	Amphotericin B, dapsone, flucytosine, pentamidine	↑ bone-marrow toxicity		CBC weekly
	Ganciclovir	↑ bone-marrow toxicity (neutropenia)	Hold zidovudine during induction therapy with ganciclovir. Reinstitute with caution during maintenance or switch to ddI/ddC.	CBC with differential 3 × weekly initially, then weekly.
	Sulfadiazine/pyrimethamine	↓ zidovudine clearance. ↑ bone-marrow toxicity; zidovudine ↓ pyrimethamine effect vs. toxoplasmosis	Consider holding zidovudine during therapy for toxoplasmosis and replacing with ddI/ddC. Folinic acid 10–50 mg daily is recommended to ↓ pyrimethamine toxicity.	CBC with differential weekly.
	TMP-SMX (trimethoprim-sulfamethoxazole, co-trimoxazole, Septra, Bactrim)	↑ anemia, neutropenia	Consider holding zidovudine during acute therapy for PCP with high-dose TMP-SMX.	CBC with differential weekly.

(Continued)

DRUGS	CONCOMITANT DRUG	COMMON SIDE EFFECTS/TOXICITY	COMMENTS	MONITORING
Antivirals Acyclovir (Zovirax)	Nephrotoxins: aminoglycosides, amphotericin B, foscarnet, pentamidine IV	Additive nephrotoxicity if combined with high-dose IV acyclovir	Cautious use of combinations is warranted.	SCr, urea 3 × weekly
	Zidovudine	↑ lethargy (case report); ? synergistic antiretroviral activity	Combination is usually well-tolerated.	
Ganciclovir (Cytovene)	Amphotericin B, dapsone, flucytosine, pentamidine IV, primaquine, pyrimethamine, TMP-SMX, trimetrexate	↑ risk of bone marrow toxicity	Cautious use of combinations is warranted.	Monitor closely for blood dyscrasias.
	ddl	*With PO ganciclovir:* ↑ ddl conc. >100%; ↓ GCV conc. 20% with sequential administration *With IV ganciclovir:* ↑ ddl conc. >70%	See ddl	See ddl
	Imipenem	↑ risk of seizures	Do not exceed 2g/day of imipenem. Dose adjust both agents in renal failure.	SCr, urea

Foscarnet (Foscavir)	Zidovudine	↑ risk of neutropenia, anemia	See zidovudine	See zidovudine
	Nephrotoxins: Pentamidine IV Acyclovir IV	Additive nephrotoxicity ↑↑ risk of ↓ Ca²⁺ & ↓ Mg²⁺ ↑ risk of nephrotoxicity	See acyclovir See pentamidine	See acyclovir See pentamidine
Antifungals Amphotericin B (Fungizone, Ambisone)	Flucytosine	↓ renal elimination of flucytosine→ ↑ flucytosine toxicity	If combination is used, flucytosine levels should be performed	SCr, urea, flucytosine levels
	Nephrotoxins Zidovudine	Additive nephrotoxicity Additive anemia	See acyclovir	See acyclovir Monitor CBC as above.
Fluconazole (Diflucan)			Fluconazole is hepatic enzyme inhibitor (less potent than ketonazole); may ↓ clearance of other metabolized agents.	
	Carbamazepine	↓ fluconazole concentrations	May have to increase dose of fluconazole.	Monitor for fluconazole efficacy.

(Continued)

DRUGS	CONCOMITANT DRUG	COMMON SIDE EFFECTS/TOXICITY	COMMENTS	MONITORING
	Nonsedating H$_1$ antagonists	Cardiac repolarization abnormalities	Caution warranted with combination. Preferable to use terfenadine or to change to sedating antihistamine.	Monitor for cardiac arrhythmias.
	Phenytoin	↑ phenytoin AUC* (75%); ↓ fluconazole concentration	May result in phenytoin toxicity and decreased fluconazole efficacy.	Monitor phenytoin & albumin levels; watch for phenytoin toxicity; monitor for fluconazole efficacy.
	Rifabutin	↑ rifabutin concentrations 80%-cases of uveitis reported	Do not exceed rifabutin 300 mg/day while on combination.	Monitor for signs and symptoms of uveitis; measure rifabutin concentrations where available.
	Rifampin	↓ fluconazole AUC (25%)	May result in decreased fluconazole efficacy.	Monitor for fluconazole efficacy.
	Sulfonylureas	↑ sulfonyurea conc. ≤100%	May ↓ blood glucose levels	Blood glucose; adjust dose prn

Theophylline		↓ theophylline metabolic clearance (15-20%)	May result in theophylline toxicity.	Monitor theophylline levels; watch for theophylline toxicity.
	Warfarin	↑ PT	Possible ↑ risk of bleeding.	Monitor PT, adjust warfarin dose as required.
Ketoconazole (Nizoral)			Ketoconazole is a potent hepatic enzyme inhibitor. Take with food if GI upset. Requires acidic media for absorption (take with orange juice or cola).	
	Antacids, ddI, H₂ antagonists, omeprazole	↓ ketoconazole bioavailability due to ↑ gastric pH	Give ketoconazole 2 hours before or after antacids and ddI. Concurrent administration with H₂ antagonists and/or omeprazole is not recommended, since absorption may be ↓↓. Consider fluconazole use in such cases.	Monitor for efficacy of ketoconazole.

(Continued)

AUC = Area under the concentration-time curve.

DRUGS	CONCOMITANT DRUG	COMMON SIDE EFFECTS/TOXICITY	COMMENTS	MONITORING
	Carbamazepine Cisapride	↓ azole concentrations QT prolongation and ventricular arrhythmias	See fluconazole Avoid combination. Consider use of other prokinetic agents.	See fluconazole
	Nonsedating H₁ antagonists	Cardiac repolarization abnormalities	Avoid with all nonsedating antihistamines. Consider combining with sedating antihistamine or using fluconazole with terfenadine.	
	Isoniazid	↑ ketoconazole metabolism	Higher doses of ketoconazole may be needed.	Monitor for efficacy of ketoconazole.
	Phenytoin	↓↑ phenytoin concentration; ↓ ketoconazole concentration	Coadministration may cause altered metabolism of one or both drugs.	Monitor serum phenytoin levels and albumin; monitor for efficacy of ketoconazole.

	Rifampin	↑ ketoconazole metab-olism; ↓ rifampin absorption	May explain apparent ketoconazole and rifampin failure. Avoid combination; consider using fluconazole or itraconazole if antifungal is required.
	Sulfonylureas	↑ sulfonylurea conc. ≤100%	See fluconazole
	Warfarin	↑ PT	See fluconazole
Itraconazole (Sporanox)			Itraconazole is a hepatic enzyme inhibitor. The capsules should be taken with food and an acidic beverage such as orange juice or Coke. The solution is best absorbed on an empty stomach.
	Antacids, ddl, H₁ antagonist, omeprazole	↓ azole bioavailability due to ↑ gastric pH	See ketoconazole
	Carbamazepine	↓ azole concentrations	See fluconazole
	Cisapride	QT prolongation and ventricular arrhythmias	See ketoconazole

(Continued)

DRUGS	CONCOMITANT DRUG	COMMON SIDE EFFECTS/TOXICITY	COMMENTS	MONITORING
	Digoxin	↑ digoxin concentrations	Predisposes to digoxin toxicity due to ↑ digoxin concentrations and ↓K$^+$.	Monitor serum digoxin concentrations and electrolytes. Watch for symptoms of digoxin toxicity.
	Nonsedating H$_1$ antagonists	Cardiac repolarization abnormalities	See ketoconazole	See ketoconazole.
	Phenytoin	↓ itraconazole conc.		Monitor for itraconazole efficacy.
	Rifampin, rifabutin	↓ itraconazole concentrations		Monitor for itraconazole efficacy.
	Sulfonylureas	↑ sulfonylurea conc. ≤100%	See fluconazole	See fluconazole
	Warfarin	↑ PT	See fluconazole	See fluconazole
Antimycobacterial Therapy				
Azithromycin (Zithromax)			Less effect on hepatic enzymes than clarithromycin. Take on an empty stomach.	

		Clarithromycin is an enzyme inhibitor.	
Clarithromycin (Biaxin)			
	Carbamazepine, theophylline	↓ carbamazepine and theophylline metabolism, resulting in ↑ conc.	Monitor levels and for symptoms of toxicity.
	Nonsedating H₁ antagonists	Cardiac repolarization abnormalities	Avoid combination. Consider use of azithromycin or a sedating antihistamine instead.
	Rifabutin	↑ rifabutin conc. 78%; ↓ clarithromycin conc. by 50%	Consider ↑ clarithromycin dose if no therapeutic response, but may ↑ rifabutin levels, which may lead to rifabutin toxicity, including uveitis. Therapeutic efficacy of clarithromycin, dose-related toxicities of rifabutin.
Clofazimine (Lamprene)	Phenytoin	↓ phenytoin concentrations	Mechanism unknown. Monitor phenytoin levels, albumin and for loss of seizure control.
Ethambutol (Myambutol, Etibi)	Aluminum salts	↓ ethambutol absorption	Separate aluminum salts from ethambutol by at least 2 hours.

(Continued)

DRUGS	CONCOMITANT DRUG	COMMON SIDE EFFECTS/TOXICITY	COMMENTS	MONITORING
Isoniazid (INH)	Aluminum salts	↓ INH absorption	Separate aluminum salts from INH by at least 2 hours.	
	Carbamazepine	↓ carbamazepine metabolism		Monitor carbamazepine levels and for symptoms of toxicity.
	Ketoconazole	↑ ketoconazole metabolism	See ketoconazole	See ketoconazole
	Phenytoin	↑ phenytoin concentrations	Probably most significant in slow metabolizers. Effect minimized with concomitant rifampin.	Monitor phenytoin, albumin and for symptoms of toxicity.
	Rifampin	↑ risk of hepatotoxicity		Monitor for signs and symptoms of hepatotoxicity.
	Sulfonylureas	Hyperglycemia	INH may lead to a loss of glucose control in patients on oral hypoglycemics.	Monitor blood glucose.

Pyrazinamide (PZA)	Rifampin	↑ rifampin metabolism (~5%)	See rifampin
Quinolones: Ciprofloxacin (Cipro) Ofloxacin (Floxin)			
	Antacids, ddI, iron, aluminum, calcium, zinc, magnesium, sucralfate, enteral feeds, vitamins with minerals	↓ quinolone absorption by ≤90% due to formation of chelation complexes with di-trivalent cations.	Ciprofloxacin is a more potent inhibitor of hepatic enzymes than ofloxacin. Best to avoid combination; if necessary, administer listed products 6 hours before or 2 hours after quinolones.	Monitor for quinolone efficacy.
	Theophylline	↑ theophylline concentrations (20%)	Enoxacin > ciprofloxacin > ofloxacin.	Monitor theophylline levels and for symptoms of toxicity. Monitor PT
	Warfarin	May ↑ PT	Few case reports.	
Rifabutin (Mycobutin)	Clarithromycin, fluconazole	↑ rifabutin concentrations	Is a less potent inducer of hepatic enzymes than rifampin. Potential uveitis; see clarithromycin and fluconazole	Monitor for dose-related rifabutin toxicity.

(Continued)

DRUGS	CONCOMITANT DRUG	COMMON SIDE EFFECTS/TOXICITY	COMMENTS	MONITORING
Rifampin (Rifadin)	Itraconazole	↓ itraconazole concentration	May require higher doses of itraconazole	Monitor for itraconazole efficacy.
	Phenytoin	May possibly ↓ phenytoin concentration	May require higher doses of phenytoin.	Monitor for phenytoin efficacy and serum concentrations.
			Rifampin is a potent hepatic enzyme inducer. Caution with contact lenses (staining).	
	Atovaquone	↓ atovaquone AUC by >50%, ↑ rifampin AUC by >30%	Potential for therapeutic failure.	Monitor for clinical efficacy with atovaquone.
	Fluconazole, ketoconazole, oral contraceptives, sulfonylureas	↑ metabolism of agents listed	Patients may require higher doses of drugs listed when coadministered with rifampin. An additional method of birth control should be considered. When treating TB, avoid combination of ketoconazole and rifampin. See ketoconazole.	Monitor for efficacy of respective agent.

Antiparasitic Agents

Atovaquone			
Phenytoin	↓ phenytoin concentration (>50%)	May need to ↑ phenytoin dose.	Monitor for breakthrough seizures.
Pyrazinamide	↑ rifampin metabolism (~5%)	Clinical significance unclear.	Monitor for efficacy of TB therapy.
Rifampin	↓ atovaquone AUC by >50%, ↑ rifampin AUC by >30%	See rifampin	See rifampin
Dapsone			
Pyrimethamine Primaquine	↑ bone marrow toxicity ↑ risk of hemolytic anemia, methemoglobinemia	See general comment for dapsone	CBC See general comment for dapsone
Rifampin	↑ dapsone clearance	Higher dapsone doses may be necessary.	Monitor for dapsone efficacy.
Trimethoprim (TMP)	↑ both dapsone and TMP conc. by approx. 40%	Consider reducing the dose of TMP in patients with baseline anemia or if anemia develops.	CBC
Zidovudine	↑ bone marrow toxicity		CBC weekly to monthly

(Continued)

DRUGS	CONCOMITANT DRUG	COMMON SIDE EFFECTS/TOXICITY	COMMENTS	MONITORING
Pentamidine IV (Pentacarinat)	Amphotericin B	↑ risk of ↓ Mg^{2+} ↑ risk of nephrotoxicity	Caution warranted with combination.	Scr, urea, electrolytes, Mg 3 × weekly
	Foscarnet	↑↑ risk of ↓ Ca^{2+} & ↓ Mg^{2+} ↑ risk of nephrotoxicity	Strongly consider alternatives before combining these drugs. Aggressive pretherapy hydration may ↓ nephrotoxicity	Scr, urea, electrolytes, Ca, Mg 3 × weekly
	Pancreatoxins	↑ risk of pancreatitis	See ddC	See ddC
Pyrimethamine (Daraprim)		Skin rash, pancytopenia	Give folinic acid 10–50mg/ day with pyrimethamine.	CBC
	Zidovudine	↓ zidovudine clearance. ↑ bone-marrow toxicity; zidovudine ↓ pyrimethamine effect vs toxoplasmosis	See zidovudine	See zidovudine
	TMP-SMX	Megaloblastic anemia, leukopenia	See TMP-SMX	See TMP-SMX
Sulfadiazine	Sulfonylureas	Decreased blood glucose	See TMP-SMX	See TMP-SMX
	Warfarin	↑ PT	See TMP-SMX	See TMP-SMX

Drug	Interacting drug	Effect	Mechanism/Comments	Monitoring
TMP-SMX (trimethoprim-sulfamethoxazole, co-trimoxazole, Septra, Bactrim)	Phenytoin	↑ phenytoin concentrations		Monitor phenytoin levels and serum albumin—modify dose accordingly.
	Pyrimethamine	Megaloblastic anemia, leukopenia	Additive inhibition of di-hydrofolate reductase. Use together in low dosages. Folinic acid should be given with pyrimethamine, but is not effective in reducing TMP-SMX hematotoxicity.	CBC with differential weekly
	Sulfonylureas	Decreased blood glucose	TMP-SMX inhibits sulfonylurea metabolic clearance	Monitor blood glucose.
	Warfarin	↑ PT	TMP-SMX inhibits warfarin metabolic clearance	Monitor PT.
Anticonvulsant Medications Phenytoin (Dilantin)			Is an enzyme inducer. Also susceptible to other inducers/inhibitors. Is protein bound; may displace other highly bound drugs.	Always check serum albumin (often ↓ in HIV) when measuring phenytoin levels.

(Continued)

DRUGS	CONCOMITANT DRUG	COMMON SIDE EFFECTS/TOXICITY	COMMENTS	MONITORING
	Chloramphenicol	↑ phenytoin concentration	Avoid chloramphenicol if possible.	Symptoms of phenytoin toxicity.
	Cimetidine	↑ phenytoin concentration (≤70%)	Effect may vary with cimetidine dose; interaction usually occurs in few days, resolves within 2 weeks of D/C cimetidine. Consider switching to other H₂ antagonists.	Symptoms of phenytoin toxicity, serum phenytoin levels.
	Clofazimine	↓ phenytoin concentration	See clofazimine	See clofazimine
	Disulfiram	↑ phenytoin concentration; symptoms of toxicity reported	Onset of interaction is rapid (≤4 hrs of first dose), resolves within 3 weeks after disulfiram D/C.	Monitor for symptoms of phenytoin toxicity; ↓ dose if necessary.
	Doxycycline	↓ doxycycline concentration	Potential therapeutic failure. May need to ↑ dose or switch to another tetracycline.	Monitor for doxycycline efficacy.

Fluconazole	↑ phenytoin AUC (75%) 75%, ↓ fluconazole concentration	See fluconazole	See fluconazole
Ketoconazole	↓↑ phenytoin concentration ↓ ketoconazole concentration	See ketoconazole	See ketoconazole
Itraconazole	↓ itraconazole concentration	See itraconazole	See itraconazole
Isoniazid	↑ phenytoin concentration	See isoniazid	See isoniazid
Methadone	↓ methadone concentration; may lead to withdrawal symptoms	Interaction usually occurs within 3–4 days of starting phenytoin. ↑ methadone dose if necessary.	Symptoms of methadone withdrawal.
Omeprazole	↑ phenytoin concentration	Adjust phenytoin dose if necessary.	Symptoms of phenytoin toxicity.
Oral contraceptives	↓ conc. of oral contraceptive	Menstrual irregularities and unplanned pregnancy may occur.	Consider alternative/additional method of contraception.
Rifabutin	Potential ↓ phenytoin concentration	See rifabutin	See rifabutin

(Continued)

DRUGS	CONCOMITANT DRUG	COMMON SIDE EFFECTS/TOXICITY	COMMENTS	MONITORING
	Rifampin	↓ phenytoin concentration (>50%)	See rifampin	See rifampin
	Serotonin reuptake inhibitors (SSRIs)	Potential ↑ phenytoin concentration	Spontaneous reports of phenytoin toxicity; may need to ↓ phenytoin dose.	Symptoms of phenytoin toxicity.
	TMP-SMX	↑ phenytoin concentration	See TMP-SMX	See TMP-SMX
	Tricyclic antidepressants (TCAs)	↓ TCA concentration	↑ metabolism of TCAs Therapeutic doses of TCAs may ↓ seizure threshold in precipitate seizures in predisposed patients.	Monitor for altered seizure activity and ↓ antidepressant effect. Measure drug levels (if available) and adjust doses if necessary.
Carbamazepine (Tegretol)	Clarithromycin	↑ carbamazepine concentration	An enzyme inducer. Also susceptible to induction/inhibition by other agents. See clarithromycin	See clarithromycin

Drug–Drug Interactions 329

Erythromycin	↑ carbamazepine concentration (>200%)	Adjust carbamazepine dose if necessary.	Symptoms of carbamazepine toxicity; obtain drug levels if available.
Fluconazole	↓ fluconazole concentration	See fluconazole	See fluconazole
Haloperidol	↓ haloperidol concentrations ≤60%	Potential clinical deterioration; ↑ dose haloperidol if necessary.	Monitor for haloperidol efficacy.
Isoniazid	↑ carbamazepine concentration	See isoniazid	See isoniazid
Methadone	↓ methadone concentration	May precipitate withdrawal; ↑ methadone dose if necessary.	Symptoms of methadone withdrawal.
Propoxyphene	↑ carbamazepine levels 200-300%	Avoid combination if possible; may need to ↓ carbamazepine dose.	Symptoms of carbamazepine toxicity.
Tricyclic antidepressants (TCAs)	Potential ↓ TCA levels	May need to ↑ TCA dose.	Monitor for altered response to TCAs whenever starting/stopping carbamazepine.

(Continued)

DRUGS	CONCOMITANT DRUG	COMMON SIDE EFFECTS/TOXICITY	COMMENTS	MONITORING
Valproic acid	Phenobarbital	↑ phenobarbital levels	Enzyme inhibitor. Highly protein bound. Via inhibition of phenobarbital metabolism. May need to ↓ phenobarbital dose.	Watch for signs or symptoms of phenobarbital toxicity.
	Phenytoin	Temporary ↑ free phenytoin levels from protein binding sites; ↑ free phenytoin followed by ↑ phenytoin clearance; thus, change in phenytoin dose not usually necessary.	Valproic acid displaces phenytoin	
Psychotropic Medications Serotonin reuptake inhibitors (SSRIs: fluoxetine, fluvoxamine, paroxetine, sertraline)			Enzyme inhibitors. Also susceptible in induction/inhibition by other drugs. Highly protein bound—may be displaced by other agents.	

Drug	Effect	Comment	Monitor
Alprazolam	↑ alprazolam concentration; ↑ psychomotor impairment	Noted with fluoxetine; may need to ↓ alprazolam dose.	Symptoms of psychomotor impairment.
Anticoagulants	Potential ↑ PT	Most marked effect with fluvoxamine; may need to adjust warfarin dose.	Monitor PT.
Barbiturates	Potential ↓ SSRI conc.	May need to ↑ SSRI dose.	Monitor therapeutic response to SSRI.
Cimetidine	↑ SSRI concentration	Substantial ↑ noted with paroxetine; use another H₂-blocker or ↓ paroxetine dose.	Symptoms of SSRI toxicity.
Dextromethorphan	↑ dextromethorphan concentration; 1 case report of hallucinations	Fluvoxamine, sertraline may be *less* potent inhibitors; consider codeine for cough suppression.	Symptoms of dextromethorphan toxicity.
Hypericin (hypericum perforatum; St. John's wort)	Potential serotonin syndrome	Hypericin acts as an MAO inhibitor. Potency may vary between products. Avoid using combination if possible.	Symptoms of serotonin syndrome.

(Continued)

DRUGS	CONCOMITANT DRUG	COMMON SIDE EFFECTS/TOXICITY	COMMENTS	MONITORING
	Lithium	Possible ↑ lithium toxicity, neurotoxicity	Use combination with caution; adjust doses as required.	CNS effects, symptoms of lithium toxicity.
	Monoamine oxidase inhibitors (MAOIs) (nonselective)	Serotonin syndrome; several fatal cases reported	Avoid concomitant use. Allow washout period of 5 half-lives (2-5 weeks) of SSRI before switching to MAOI.	Symptoms of serotonin syndrome.
	Neuroleptics	↑ neuroleptic concentration	↑ risk extrapyramidal side effects (EPS)	EPS symptoms.
	Phenytoin	Potential ↑ phenytoin concentration	See phenytoin	See phenytoin
	Theophylline	↑ theophylline concentration	Severe theophylline toxicity reported with fluvoxamine; other SSRIs may be less potent; ↓ theophylline dose if necessary.	Symptoms of theophylline toxicity.
	TCAS, trazodone	↑ TCA/trazodone concentration	Sertraline may be less likely to inhibit metabolism than other SSRIs. When adding SSRI to TCAS, should ↓ TCA dose by at least 50–67%.	Symptoms of TCA toxicity.

Tricyclic antidepressants (TCAs: amitriptyline, nortriptyline, imipramine, desipramine, etc.)			
	Carbamazepine	Potential ↓ TCA concentration	Susceptibel to induction/inhibition by other agents. See carbamazepine	Serum levels may be available. See carbamazepine
	Cimetidine	↑ TCA concentration, ↑ risk anticholinergic side effects	Other H₂-blockers less likely to interact.	Monitor for TCA toxicity.
	Hypericin	Potential hypertensive crisis	Hypericin acts as an MAOI. See MAOI below.	See MAOI below.
	MAOI	Hypertensive crisis, possible serotonergic reaction	Use combination with caution. OK to add MAOI to TCA, but cannot add TCA to MAOI; need 2 week MAOI washout period.	BP, signs/symptoms of serotonin syndrome
	RIMA (moclobemide)	Serotonin syndrome	Avoid concomitant use.	Signs/symptoms of serotonin syndrome.
	Phenytoin	↓ TCA concentration	See phenytoin	See phenytoin
	SSRIs	↑ TCA concentration	See SSRIs	See SSRIs
	Heavy smoking	↓ TCA concentration	May get subtherapeutic level at regular doses.	Obtain TCA serum level if no response at normal dose.

(Continued)

DRUGS	CONCOMITANT DRUG	COMMON SIDE EFFECTS/TOXICITY	COMMENTS	MONITORING
Lithium (Li)	Anticonvulsants	Potentiation of neurotoxicity.	May occur at normal levels of both drugs. Consider lowering dose or stopping one drug.	↑ ataxia, dizziness, tremor, muscle weakness
	Antidepressants	Potentiation of neurological effects.	Consider lowering dose of antidepressant.	Watch for aggravation of lithium tremor.
	Diuretics	↑ Li conc. via ↑ reabsorption of Na/Li in proximal tubule	Well documented with thiazides; may need to ↓ Li dose by 40%; initiate thiazide gradually. Interaction less significant with loop/K-sparing diuretics; caution recommended.	Signs/symptoms of dehydration, lithium toxicity. Obtain Li level.
	Neuroleptics	Potentiation of neurotoxicity. Consider lowering dose of neuroleptic.	Consider lowering dose of neuroleptic.	Watch for ↑ EPS, confusion, ataxia.
	NSAIDs	↑ Li conc. 30–60% by ↓ renal clearance (via renal prostaglandin inhibition)	Occurs gradually over several days; elderly at ↑ risk. No effect with ASA, sulindac.	Obtain Li level; watch for signs/symptoms of Li toxicity.

Haloperidol (Haldol)	Nephrotoxins	↑ Li conc. via ↓ renal clearance	Adjust Li dose if necessary.	Monitor renal function, Li levels.
	Carbamazepine	↓ haloperidol conc. ≤60%	See carbamazepine	See carbamazepine
	Lithium	↑ risk neurotoxicity	See lithium	See lithium
	SSRIs	↑ haloperidol concentrations	See SSRIs	See SSRIs
Methylphenidate (Ritalin)	Pressor agents, MAOIs, hypericin	↑ risk hypertension	Potential enzyme inhibitor. Sympathomimetic effects at high doses. Use combination with caution.	Monitor BP, HR, etc.
	Oral anticoagulants, anticonvulsants, TCAs	Possible ↑ conc. of agents in column 2.	Metabolism of listed agents may be inhibited by concurrent use of methylphenidate. Adjust doses if required.	Serum levels of listed agents.

Appendix 4: Drug–Food Interactions

Michelle Foisy, Pharm.D.

Alice Tseng, Pharm.D.

DRUG	TAKE WITH FOOD	TAKE ON EMPTY STOMACH	TAKE REGARDLESS OF FOOD	COMMENTS
Antiretroviral Agents				
ddC (dideoxycytidine, zalcitabine, HIVID)			X	
ddI (dideoxyinosine, didanosine, Videx)		X		Requires a basic media for absorption. Contains Mg^{2+} & Al^{3+} as buffers.
d4T (stavudine)			X	
3TC (lamivudine)			X	
Zidovudine (AZT, Retrovir)	Avoid taking with fatty meals. Food may help to ↓ nausea.	Best absorbed if taken on an empty stomach (if patient can tolerate this).		Take in an upright position with a full glass of water to minimize risk of esophageal ulceration.

(Continued)

DRUG	TAKE WITH FOOD	TAKE ON EMPTY STOMACH	TAKE REGARDLESS OF FOOD	COMMENTS
PCP Therapy				
TMP-SMX (trimethoprim-sulfamethoxazole, cotrimoxazole, Septra, Bactrim)			X	Take with a large glass of water each time to ensure adequate hydration.
Dapsone (Avlosulfone)			X	
Trimethoprim (Proloprim)			X	
Clindamycin + Primaquine			X	Take with food to minimize GI upset.
Atovaquone (Mepron)	Take with fatty foods to enhance absorption.			
Antivirals				
Acyclovir (Zovirax)			X	Take large oral doses (i.e., 800 mg 5x/d) with plenty of water to ensure adequate hydration.
Ganciclovir PO (Cytovene)	X (to ↑ absorption)			

Antifungals				Comments
Fluconazole (Diflucan)			X	
Flucytosine (Ancotil)			X	Each dose should be taken over a 15 minute period with food to minimize GI upset.
Ketoconazole (Nizoral)	X			Requires an acidic media for absorption. To enhance absorption take with an acidic beverage such as orange juice, cranberry juice, or cola. See Appendix 3.
Itraconazole (Sporanox)	X (capsules)	X (solution)		See ketoconazole (applies to capsules only). See Appendix 3.
Nystatin (Mycostatin)		X		Avoid eating for at least 30 minutes after treatment to ↑ mucosal contact time. Rinse mouth well prior to swishing; retain in mouth for several minutes and then swallow.

(Continued)

DRUG	TAKE WITH FOOD	TAKE ON EMPTY STOMACH	TAKE REGARDLESS OF FOOD	COMMENTS
Clotrimazole troches and vaginal tablets (Canesten, Myclo, Mycelex) Amphotericin B troches, solution (Fungizone)		X		See nystatin. Allow troches or vaginal tablets to dissolve in mouth.
Toxoplasmosis Therapy				
Sulfadiazine			X	Take with a large glass of water each time to ensure adequate hydration.
Pyrimethamine (Daraprim)			X	
Folinic acid (leucovorin)			X	
Clindamycin			X	Take with food to minimize GI upset.

Antimycobacterials

Quinolones

Drug			Notes
Ciprofloxacin (Cipro), Ofloxacin (Floxin)		X	Minimize caffeine intake. Milk, milk products, enteral feeds, nutritional supplements (e.g., Boost, Resource), and mineral supplements may ↓ absorption. See Appendix 3.
Azithromycin (Zithromax)	X		
Clarithromycin (Biaxin)		X	
Clofazimine (Lamprene)	X (may ↑ absorption)		
Cycloserine (Seromycin)		X	Take with food to minimize GI upset.
Ethambutol (Myambutol, Etibi)		X	See Appendix 3.
Ethionamide (Trecator)		X	Take with food to minimize GI upset.

(Continued)

DRUG	TAKE WITH FOOD	TAKE ON EMPTY STOMACH	TAKE REGARDLESS OF FOOD	COMMENTS
Isoniazid (INH)		X (may ↑ absorption)		See Appendix 3.
Para-aminosalicylic acid (PAS)	X			Take with food to minimize GI upset.
Pyrazinamide (PZA, Tebrazid)			X	
Rifabutin (Mycobutin)			X	If GI effects, divide dose: 150 mg at breakfast and at dinner.
Rifampin (Rifadin)		X (may ↑ absorption)		
Other Antibiotics				
Amoxicillin (Amoxil)			X	
Ampicillin (Penbritin)		X		
Cefaclor (Ceclor)			X	
Cephalexin (Keflex)			X	

Cloxacillin (Orbenin)	X		
Cefixime (Suprax)		X	
Cefuroxime axetil (Ceftin)	X (↑ absorption)		
Doxycycline (Vibramycin)		X	Take with food to minimize GI upset. Take in an upright position to minimize esophageal ulceration. Can take doxycycline with milk and milk products with minimal effect on absorption. Should take at least 2 hours before or 3–4 hours after drugs containing ditrivalent cations (Al^{3+}, Ca^{2+}, Fe^{2+}, Mg^{2+}, Zn^{2+}).
Erythromycin base (Erythromid)	X		

(Continued)

DRUG	TAKE WITH FOOD	TAKE ON EMPTY STOMACH	TAKE REGARDLESS OF FOOD	COMMENTS
Erythromycin base		X		Take at least 30 minutes before eating. Do not crush or chew.
Enteric-coated tablets (Erybid, Eryc, PCE) (E-Mycin)			X	Do not crush or chew.
Erythromycin stearate (Erythrocin)		X		
Erythromycin estolate (Ilosone)			X	
Erythromycin ethylsuccinate (EES)	X (may ↑ absorption)			
Iodoquinol (Diodoquin)			X	Take with food to minimize GI upset.
Metronidazole (Flagyl)			X	Take with food to minimize GI upset. Avoid taking with alcohol and for 48 hours after D/C metronidazole.

Drug			
Paromomycin (Humatin)		X	Take with food to minimize GI upset.
Penicillin V (Pen-Vee, PVF-K)		X	See doxycycline. In addition, administer tetracycline at least 1–2 hours apart from milk and milk products.
Penicillin G (Megacillin)	X		
Tetracycline (Tetracyn)	X		
Thiabendazole (Mintezol)		X	Take with food to minimize GI upset.
Miscellaneous			
Calcium carbonate (Os-Cal, Caltrate)	X (↑ absorption)		
Carbamazepine (Tegretol)		X	Take with food to minimize GI upset.
Iron (Ferrous sulfate, Slow-Fe)	Food may ↓ GI upset.		Best absorbed on an empty stomach. Do not crush or chew slow-release preparations.

(Continued)

DRUG	TAKE WITH FOOD	TAKE ON EMPTY STOMACH	TAKE REGARDLESS OF FOOD	COMMENTS
Narcotic analgesics. NSAIDs	X		X	
Omeprazole (Losec)		X		Take in the morning if possible. Do not crush or chew.
Phenytoin (Dilantin)			X (but not with enteral supplements)	Give 2 hours before or after enteral supplements. Take at hs to minimize daytime drowsiness.
Pyridoxine (Vitamin B₆)			X	
Sucralfate (Sulcrate)		X		Take 30 min–1 hour before meals. Avoid antacids within 30 min. Contains Al^{3+}; caution with interacting agents.

Index

Note: Page numbers in *italics* refer to illustrations; those followed by t refer to tables.